M000073399

The New Science of Psychedelics

"David Jay Brown's book is a persuasive and necessary argument as we collectively move toward the mainstreaming of psychedelics and face the unique survival challenges of the twenty-first century. This is an outstanding book to read and share widely."

RICK DOBLIN, FOUNDER OF THE MULTIDISCIPLINARY ASSOCIATION FOR PSYCHEDELIC STUDIES (MAPS)

"This is a simply splendid book! David Brown is a leading-edge activist, explorer, and philosopher who has blended an astounding number of personal experiences as well as commentaries from amazing people into a narrative that goes well beyond other books about psychedelics. He reevaluates not only the well-known areas of healing, psychotherapy, creativity, and spirituality but also extends his wise deliberations and deep explorations into areas that most of us still shy away from—freely discussing alien encounters, psychedelic sex, mixing and matching various substances, parapsychology, consciousness after death, and more—drawing on his own extensive voyages and exploration for telling examples. He is unafraid to explore the dark sides of his own personality as well as his joys as needed to illuminate challenging aspects of the multifaceted psychedelic universe."

JAMES FADIMAN, PH.D., AUTHOR OF *THE PSYCHEDELIC EXPLORER'S GUIDE*

"David Jay Brown writes it all up in a sure hand with a flare appropriate to the subject matter so that the reader is as much entertained as informed."

R.U. Sirius, author of *Everybody Must Get Stoned*

"If your taste is for paradigm busting, you'll find lots of food for thought in *The New Science of Psychedelics*. On the menu are parapsychology, unexplained phenomena, strange powers, scientific mysteries, confounding conventional science, odd animal behavior, morphic fields, the Gaia hypothesis, alien beings, entities, forbidden knowledge, kundalini, survival after death, and more."

Thomas B. Roberts, author of
The Psychedelic Future of the Mind

"*The New Science of Psychedelics* is a knockout! David Jay Brown tackles the touchy topic of 'sex on drugs' with the wisdom of hands-on experience, an expanded mind, and the ability to get into deep places. This book reads like an honest, intimate love letter!"

Annie Sprinkle, Ph.D., sex worker turned
EcoSexologist and coauthor of *Urban Tantra:
Sacred Sex for the Twenty-First Century*

"Dave's particular mixture of youthful curiosity, honest skepticism, and appetite for adventure remind me of Tom Sawyer. Reading this book is like riding a raft with Tom down the psychedelic Mississippi. You meet anew all the famous natives who live along its shores—Tim Leary, Robert Anton Wilson, John Lilly, and many others. This book captures both the peculiar terrors and the deep delights these mind-altering substances can induce. A no-nonsense personal exploration of a controversial area of scientific research recounted in a light and engaging manner."

Nick Herbert, author of
Quantum Reality: Beyond the New Physics

The New Science of
Psychedelics

At the Nexus of Culture, Consciousness, and Spirituality

David Jay Brown

Park Street Press
Rochester, Vermont • Toronto, Canada

Park Street Press
One Park Street
Rochester, Vermont 05767
www.ParkStPress.com

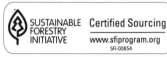

Text stock is SFI certified

Park Street Press is a division of Inner Traditions International

Copyright © 2013 by David Jay Brown

All rights reserved. No part of this book may be reproduced or utilized in
any form or by any means, electronic or mechanical, including photocopying,
recording, or by any information storage and retrieval system, without permission
in writing from the publisher.

Library of Congress Cataloging-in-Publication Data
Brown, David Jay.
  The new science of psychedelics : at the nexus of culture, consciousness, and
spirituality / David Jay Brown.
      pages cm
  Includes index.
  Summary: "What does the future hold for humanity, and can psychedelics help
take us there?"—Provided by publisher.
  ISBN 978-1-59477-492-8 (pbk.) — ISBN 978-1-62055-142-4 (e-book)
  1. Hallucinogenic drugs. 2. Consciousness. I. Title.
  BF209.H34N49 2013
  154.4—dc23
                                                                    2012040639

Printed and bound in the United States by Lake Book Manufacturing, Inc.
The text stock is SFI certified. The Sustainable Forestry Initiative® program
promotes sustainable forest management.

10 9 8 7 6 5 4 3 2 1

Text design by Virginia Scott Bowman and layout by Brian Boynton
This book was typeset in Garamond Premier Pro with Helvetica Neue as a display
typeface

To send correspondence to the author of this book, mail a first-class letter to the
author c/o Inner Traditions • Bear and Company, One Park Street, Rochester, VT
05767, and we will forward the communication, or contact the author directly at
www.mavericksofthemind.com.

*For all of the psychedelic agents
working to help raise consciousness,
in this universe and elsewhere*

Contents

Acknowledgments

I've thought about writing this book for many years and was glad to finally be given the opportunity. Countless people contributed to making this book what it is. I'd like to extend my deepest gratitude to all of the people who have allowed me to interview them throughout my career. Many of these busy people gave me their precious time, much of it when I was still young and inexperienced, and for these valuable opportunities I will be forever grateful.

I would like to extend my sincere appreciation to the following individuals for their generous contributions and valuable support: Carolyn Mary Kleefeld, Jon Graham, Arleen Margulis, Goo Bear, Jacob Andrade, Danielle Bohmer, Danelle Benari, Amanda Rose Loveland, Meriana Dinkova, Lily Ross, Sara Huntley, Willow Aryn Dellinger, Jessi Daichman, Serena Watman, Buck Noe, Sara Mokhtari-Fox, Selina Reddan, Veronika King, Jesse Ray Houts, Audreanne Rivka Sheehan, Patricia Holt, Linda Parker, Chanc VanWinkle Orzell, Erica B. Robinson, Denis Berry, Zach Leary, Maria Grusauskas, Rebecca McClen Novick, Annie Sprinkle, Kelly Hollerbach, Heather Goldstein Greenberg, Brandi Goldstein, Geoffrey and Valerie Goldstein, Nese Lisa Senol, Ralph Abraham, Rupert Sheldrake, Louise Reitman, Sammie and Tudie, Rob Brezsny, Rick Doblin, Amy Barnes Excolere, Sherry Hall, Suzie Wouk, Sherri Paris, Robert Forte, Valerie Leveroni Corral, David Wayne Dunn, Robin Rae and Brummbaer, Deed DeBruno,

Randy Baker, Richard Goldberg, Steven Ray Brown, B'anna Federico, Anna Damoth, Sandy Oppenheim, Lorey Capelli, Dana Peleg, Mimi Peleg, Bethan Carter, Robert J. Barnhart, Al Brown, Cheryle and Gene Goldstein, Dina Meyer, Bernadette Wilson, Nick Herbert, Damon Orion, Ian Koslow, Ralph Metzner, Erin Jarvis, Jody Lombardo, Erica Ansberry, Jessica Ansberry-Gagnon, Maria Ramirez, Rob Bryanton, Cliff Pickover, R.U. Sirius, James Fadiman, Linda D'Amato, Nathan West, and Paula Rae Mellard.

Special thanks to the Group Mind, my worldwide network of Internet friends, who inform me about new scientific developments, support my work, share their creative talents, and challenge my ideas. I am most grateful for everyone's contributions and communications.

DISCLAIMER

The information in this book is provided for informational and educational purposes only. The author does not in any way endorse the illegal use of psychedelic drugs.

NOTE TO READERS

Unless otherwise noted, all of the quotes in this volume came from personal interviews that I conducted. The complete interviews can be found in my books *Mavericks of the Mind, Voices from the Edge, Conversations on the Edge of the Apocalypse, Mavericks of Medicine,* and on my website: www.mavericksofthemind.com.

Introduction

Awakening from My Slumber and Recognizing My Preprogrammed Robotic Nature

In this book we'll be exploring a wide array of unorthodox ideas about the evolution of consciousness and the future. *The New Science of Psychedelics* contains a collection of fascinating anecdotes from my many interviews with accomplished iconic thinkers and discussions on how these interactions interfaced with the ideas, insights, and revelations from my numerous psychedelic experiences.

My career as an interviewer, science writer, scientific researcher, and science-fiction author has been inseparably linked with my thirty-three years of experimentation with psychedelic drugs and hallucinogenic plants. The areas that I was inspired to research, the subjects that I was motivated to write about, the people I chose to interview, and the questions I decided to ask them have all been thoroughly influenced by my regular and disciplined use of cannabis, LSD, psilocybin, MDMA, DMT, salvia, and other psychedelic sacraments.

Since 1989 I've been interviewing some of the most thought-provoking thinkers on the planet, with a special interest in how psychedelics have affected their work. In *The New Science of Psychedelics,* I alternate between describing my psychedelic experiences and my interview encounters, quoting from the many dozens of in-depth interviews that I have conducted over the years, in order to shed some light on the mysteries that can occur during a psychedelic journey.

In the book I quote from my interviews with luminaries such as Terence McKenna, Robert Anton Wilson, Timothy Leary, John Lilly, Allen Ginsberg, Jerry Garcia, Ram Dass, Noam Chomsky, George Carlin, Deepak Chopra, Ray Kurzweil, Andrew Weil, Jack Kevorkian, Edgar Mitchell, Albert Hofmann, Stanislav Grof, Joan Halifax, Alex Grey, H. R. Giger, Simon Posford, and Rupert Sheldrake. Some of the varied topics explored in the book include the interface between science and spirituality, lucid dreaming, time travel, morphic field theory, alternative science, optimal health, what happens to consciousness after death, encounters with nonhuman beings, the future evolution of our species, and how psychedelics affect creativity.

TRANSCENDENTAL MEDITATION

My interest in exploring altered states of consciousness grew out of a childhood fascination with science fiction, the occult, and unexplained phenomena. This interest in the mysterious aspects of reality and my own mind—as well as a desire to calm my mind, do better and improve my reading comprehension skills in school, and explore the untapped potential of my brain—led me to learn how to meditate when I was fourteen years old and a sophomore in high school.

I convinced my mom to spend $50 in 1974 so I could learn the transcendental meditation (TM) technique. I participated in a private ceremony with a "certified TM instructor," where I was given a personal mantra, which I was told to never, ever reveal to anyone else. I kept the mantra a secret for about twenty-five years before revealing it to others, and I haven't noticed any difference in my meditations since doing so. When I interviewed TM expert Peter McWilliams in 1999, I told him my mantra, and he said that it wasn't even one of the official TM mantras. Nonetheless, it has always worked for me, so now I'm passing along this magic mantra to you. Here it is: *ee-ma*.

One repeats this mantra silently in one's mind over and over, while sitting quietly with closed eyes in a peaceful environment. Whenever one stops repeating the mantra and starts thinking thoughts, it's time to start repeating the mantra again. It's that simple. With time, the mantra is repeated more and more, and thinking diminishes. This is what I learned for $50. The quasimystical ceremony, which occurred before an altar with religious objects and burning candles, undoubtedly enhanced the initial effect, but I'm sure that I could have just as easily learned the technique from reading a few sentences in a book. It's not terribly complicated, but it does take practice to master.

I began practicing TM religiously as a young teenager, sitting alone in my bedroom twice a day for twenty minutes with the door locked, while I silently repeated the mantra *ee-ma* in my head. By occupying the language/speech/thinking center of my mind with a repeating mantra, I found that my sense of awareness was liberated into a more peaceful space—one that transcended my conventional thinking process. In addition to making me a more peaceful and less anxious person, it really did improve my reading comprehension skills.

But, more important, meditation became an especially useful skill once I began to experiment with cannabis and other mind-expanding substances. Like the many Hindu sadhus before me, I found that cannabis and meditation went extremely well together and that the sacred plant enhanced my ability to transcend conceptual or verbal awareness.

Meditation also became an essential tool once I began to explore the far reaches of hyperspace with psychedelics. Whenever I ran into difficult psychological terrain on my psychedelic journeys I was always glad that I knew how to meditate when the energies became too overwhelming to process or understand. This eventually led to my realization that all spiritual practices appear to work best when combined with psychedelics.

DJB MEETS THC

My interest in meditation and the writings of Robert Anton Wilson led me to experiment with the cognitive-changing, sensory-enhancing properties of cannabis. In 1976 I purchased a small quantity of the illegal herb from a fellow student in my art class, and I picked up a small pipe with a wooden bowl at my local mall. I tried smoking the condensed, dried brown buds three times in the pipe without any noticeable effect. Then, on the fourth try, it finally worked.

I was taking tokes from my pipe in an extra bedroom, downstairs in the home that I grew up in, while my mother spoke on the phone upstairs in the kitchen. I was listening to her voice and laughter seep through the ceiling, and it seemed to be unusually interesting for some reason—dreamlike and amusing—almost like a parody or as if she were speaking in a cartoon. I was hearing these archetypal and strangely humorous qualities in my mom's voice when I suddenly realized that I was totally and completely stoned. I found the perceptual shifts, cognitive changes, and sensory enhancement that cannabis brought to be absolutely delightful, and I marveled at everything around me.

Getting high for the first time felt like being let in on a great cosmic secret. As Timothy Leary exclaimed about his first cannabis experience, "Wow. How long has this been going on?" I was astonished by my own thoughts, and my imagination became greatly enhanced. At times it became hard to determine if what I was seeing was really there or not. I saw ghostly images of my dead grandfather and dead uncle, standing together, looking at me from the foot of the bed. A translucent genie wrapped in folded cloth swam out of the heating vent as the heater came on, and spoke with the air-blowing sound of the heater, saying, "I've come to soothe you." The *oo* in *soothe* was drawn out into a long, trance-inducing auditory experience that resonated with the sound of the heater.

I soon became ravenously hungry but was far too nervous about being stoned in front of my mom, so I waited. After my mom left the kitchen I cautiously made a heroic climb up the Mt. Everest–size staircase and discovered that the coast was clear. I sat down at the kitchen table with a bowl of Kellogg's Rice Krispies and a container of cow's milk. For around thirty minutes I sat there in absolute divine bliss, eating bowl after bowl of Rice Krispies. They were the most incredibly delicious Rice Krispies I had tasted in my entire life, and I just couldn't get enough of them. It was a completely magical experience, sitting there at the kitchen table, eating a sublimely delicious cereal—that spoke to me about the secrets of existence in its snapping, popping, and crackling language—while the elves on the glowing box smiled at me.

Then afterward I went to lie down on my bed, closed my eyes, and started seeing visions. Dreamlike images shifted before my eyes, and this was my favorite aspect of the experience. I lay there for around an hour before falling asleep, watching the fascinating imagery flow behind my eyes with utter astonishment.

After that fateful day I first got high, I began using cannabis regularly by the time I was fifteen Now, more than three decades later, I continue to ingest cannabis, almost daily. I consider it one of my greatest allies, and it has been an especially wonderful addition on my psychedelic journeys with other substances.

Cannabis opens my senses. It greatly enhances my sensitivity to all forms of sensory stimulation—taste, smell, vision, touch, hearing. Music, food, sex, massage, art, film, and television all become enhanced with new dimensions, and one can become completely immersed in cultural creations as though they are real. Movies take on mythic and archetypal qualities. Every pleasurable sensation is experienced as pure, heavenly bliss. Colors become subjectively brighter, humor becomes more amusing, and music takes on more depth and texture as one discovers additional levels of auditory detail within it.

Thoughts and mental imagery become much more fluid under the influence of cannabis, and there is an increased propensity for insights into one's life and revelations into the nature of reality. It helps to raise my spirits when I'm feeling down, and it allows me to see my life from a new perspective, which I find both sacred and invaluable. It also helps to bring my body into a state of homeostasis—physical and mental balance—and it allows me to experience euphoria, bliss, and pain relief without any side effects.

I've come to use cannabis predominantly when I write and find it to be an essential part of my creative process. I follow Timothy Leary's suggestion: "If you write straight, edit stoned, and if you write stoned, edit straight." Whenever I work on a piece of writing I alternate between editing the piece while under the influence of cannabis and not. I find that this process allows me to see the work from multiple perspectives that synergize with one another, and I enjoy doing this immensely.

Robert Anton Wilson told me that he works in a similar fashion. He said:

> I have always had strong tendencies toward compulsive rewriting, polishing, refining, etc., and marijuana has intensified that. In fact, these days I seldom stop fine-tuning my prose until editors remind me about deadlines. As Paul Valery said, "A work of art is never completed, only abandoned," and I regard even my nonfiction as a kind of art.

HOW DOES CANNABIS BOOST CREATIVITY?

For many years numerous highly acclaimed artists, scientists, writers, musicians, and creative people of all sorts have claimed that cannabis holds enormous potential to enhance creativity and inspire the imagination. New scientific studies are beginning to confirm these claims, and researchers are starting to understand the psychological mechanisms behind how cannabis can improve the creative process.

There's a common myth, perpetuated by the mainstream media,

that people often mistakenly think that they're brilliant and creative while under the influence of cannabis only to find that their creations are worthless or that their insights are meaningless nonsense when they return to normal everyday consciousness.

The late astronomer Carl Sagan described this best in an essay that he wrote for Lester Grinspoon's book *Marihuana Reconsidered*. Sagan wrote:

> There is a myth about such highs: the user has an illusion of great insight, but it does not survive scrutiny in the morning. I am convinced that this is an error, and that the compelling insights achieved when high are real insights; the main problem is putting these insights in a form acceptable to the quite different self that we are when we're down the next day.

I agree with Sagan. So let's dispel this pervasive myth about cannabis right now by taking the many anecdotal reports to heart and looking at what the scientific studies have to say. From Charles Baudelaire to George Carlin, Shakespeare to Carl Sagan, Louis Armstrong to Jack Nicholson, the list of accomplished creative people who have claimed a positive influence from their use of cannabis is truly impressive. I've personally spoken with many accomplished people who made claims about how essential cannabis was for their creative process. For example, when I interviewed the late comedian George Carlin, he told me:

> Pot . . . changed my thinking. It fostered offbeat thinking. . . . Then it changed my comedy . . . I became more myself. The comedy became more personal, therefore more political, and therefore more successful. . . . So, suddenly, I also became materially successful. People started buying albums. I had four Gold albums in a row.

Brian Wilson of the Beach Boys said to *Rolling Stone* magazine that marijuana "helped" him write Pet Sounds, which was ranked by the magazine as the second greatest album of all time. Anecdotes about cannabis and creativity abound, but what does the scientific research say?

The Beckley Foundation—a nonprofit organization in England that supports pioneering, multidisciplinary research with cannabis and psychedelic drugs—funded a study by neuroscience researchers Valerie Curran and Celia Morgan at the University College London in 2012 that studied the effects of cannabis on creativity, and the results indicate that cannabis does indeed have a positive influence on the subject's creative performance.

Another study conducted by Celia Morgan and her colleagues in 2010 at University College London looked at how cannabis intoxication enhanced the effects of semantic priming, in which the activation of one word allows people to react more quickly to related words and to see more connections between words. One way that creativity can be described is the ability to find novel connections between different concepts. The study found that subjects linked distantly related words and concepts significantly quicker when they were high than when they weren't. This hyperpriming, as the researchers called it, is evidence that the flow of loose associations that cannabis users report is indeed real and not an illusion, as some skeptics have claimed.

Additionally, research by Xia Zhang and colleagues at Saskatchewan University demonstrates that THC (the primary psychoactive component of the cannabis plant) can spur neurogenesis, or new brain-cell formation, which is precisely the opposite of what government propaganda has been telling us for years—that cannabis kills brain cells. This research relates to our understanding of neuroplasticity—how the brain can reorganize neural pathways and rewire itself in order to become more efficient at processing information. We now know that the brain is continually rewiring itself and that it's always possible to grow new brain cells and learn new skills, which may play a role in creative thinking.

Cannabis has the effect of slightly increasing alpha-wave activity in the brain and increasing blood flow into the right hemisphere, which is associated with holistic, nonlinear thought. Alpha waves and right-brain thinking are generally associated with meditative and relaxed states of consciousness, which are, in turn, often associated with creativity. The link between psychedelics and creativity will be explored in more detail later in this book.

Although I stopped smoking cannabis regularly in my midthirties, because the smoke began to hurt my lungs, I have remained faithful to my green goddess. Since I stopped smoking I've been largely eating the sacred herb and find it much more psychedelic this way. I prefer making my cannabis edibles out of finely crushed organic cannabis leaf and natural peanut butter. I spread the cannabis–peanut butter mix on a cracker and bake it in the oven at 290 degrees for 30 minutes. I've used cannabis this way for creativity, as an imagination enhancer, as well as an antidepressant, a sexual enhancer, a sacrament, and a way to relax and relieve anxiety, reflect, and connect with the deeper aspects of myself and nature.

DISCOVERING THE SECRET ROOM

When I was in my early teens, not long after my parents got divorced, my dad moved out, and I started smoking cannabis, I discovered a secret room hidden in my house that I never knew existed before. The entrance to the doorless, windowless room was hidden in the back of a long walk-in closet, which was covered by a stack of old dusty boxes. While curiously rummaging around the closet one day, I discovered that behind the boxes was a small rectangular square sliced into the wall. The sliced square was still embedded in the wall, but the wooden-plaster rectangle easily pushed right through. Behind the hole in the wall was a small space under the staircase, where my dad had apparently stored some of his valuables before moving out.

I got a flashlight and climbed inside the small, rectangular hole in the wall, like I was entering a portal into another dimension or the enchanted cave of wonder from Aladdin's magic lamp. I was astonished to discover that there was a hidden room under the staircase, and it soon became a place for my younger brother and me to hang out whenever we wanted some extra privacy. My brother and I hung up psychedelic posters on the walls of the small room, lit candles, and often got stoned on cannabis together in there. It was our private world, and we didn't reveal our knowledge of the secret chamber to our mom for many years, not until long after we'd both moved out.

I learned from reading the works of the late psychologist Carl Jung that my real-life discovery was unusually similar to an archetypal dream that many adolescents frequently have. It's common for young teenagers to dream that they discover a secret room in their home that they never knew existed before, perhaps as a symbolic metaphor for entering a new stage of life or finding a hidden chamber in one's mind. I had recurring dreams as a small child where I would discover a magical passageway in the back of my bedroom closet, but actually discovering a secret room in the home where I grew up—right as I was entering adolescence and first experimenting with altered states of consciousness—seems rather uncanny to me.

However, this was merely the beginning of the many weird synchronicities and strange events that have become a regular part of my life, which is why I try to follow the valuable suggestion of my late friend neuroscientist John C. Lilly to "always expect the unexpected."

Over the years I've discovered many "secret rooms" in my mind—previously unknown brain circuits and neural programs hidden in my brain—while on LSD and other psychedelics. Once activated, these hidden neural programs seem fully complete, as though they were designed to be there for a particular purpose by some higher intelligence. As the late psychologist William James famously wrote in *The Varieties of the Religious Experience*:

Our normal waking consciousness, rational consciousness as we call it, is but one special type of consciousness, whilst all about it, parted from it by the filmiest of screens, there lie potential forms of consciousness entirely different. . . . We may go through life without suspecting their existence; but apply the requisite stimulus, and at a touch they are there in all their completeness, definite types of mentality which probably somewhere have their field of application and adaptation. No account of the universe in its totality can be final which leaves these other forms of consciousness quite disregarded.

These secret brain circuits and neural programs appear to be genetically wired into us, and turning them on for the first time is similar to discovering programs inside of one's computer that one didn't know was there.

I owned a MacBook laptop computer for around a year before I discovered the Time Machine program that was installed in it. Once I hooked up an external hard drive to the computer the Time Machine program was activated, and my computer screen suddenly shrank and dropped into a metaspace behind my virtual desktop. On my monitor a long row of computer desktops, arranged by date, appeared to be trailing behind it into outer space. I swear it seemed like smoking salvia or DMT for the first time. I thought, *Wow. I never knew my computer could do this!* This experience seemed analogous to me with regard to how new states of consciousness sometimes appear after taking psychedelics. You never know what you might find in your own brain.

DJB MEETS LSD

I tried LSD for the first time when I was sixteen years old. My curiosity to engage in this illegal form of self-exploration arose from several intersecting factors. In my high school health class I was told that LSD made people see new, never-before-seen colors, which was supposed to frighten me but instead fascinated me. I also noticed that some of the smartest and funniest kids at school were using acid, and they seemed anything but brain damaged to me. Additionally, since I was a child I had always been interested in unusual states of consciousness, and my experiments with meditation and marijuana helped to enhance this curiosity. So after watching a close friend enjoy his first LSD trip, and noting that he appeared to retain his sanity, despite all his uncontrollable laughter, I decided to give it a try.

One night during the 1977 school year, in the suburbs of central New Jersey, I swallowed a tiny purple microdot, about the size of a pinhead, that probably contained around 100 micrograms of LSD. My friends hung out with me for a few hours after I took it, but I didn't feel anything unusual. So after about three hours my friends left, and I went bed. Then it began to hit me. The first thing I noticed was that the walls in my room appeared to be breathing. My bedroom walls began to expand and contract in organic rhythms, mirroring my own breath, and I became frightened that I was losing my mind. I had heard that people can forget who they are on LSD, so as my anxiety began to escalate I started repeating my name and address over and over in my head, like a mantra, so I wouldn't forget who I was.

"My name is David Jay Brown. I live at 16 Lee Way, Somerville, New Jersey. My name is David Jay Brown . . ." I silently repeated over and over again, with increasing difficulty. My ego was rapidly dissolving, my sense of self was expanding, and I was desperately (and, in retrospect, comically) trying to hold on tight to the gooey remains of my melting ego, as my mind spilled out of my head and began to fill the room. I closed my eyes and was astonished by the colorful morphing visions that appeared within me. Terrified beyond words that I had permanently damaged my brain and that I was going insane, I also realized that if I could possibly paint onto canvas the extraordinary imagery that I was seeing behind my closed eyes, I would be the greatest artist who ever lived.

But the fear of losing my mind became too powerful, and as the effects intensified I vowed to flush all the cannabis in my closet down the toilet in the morning and to never do LSD ever again. With no previous training in shamanism or mysticism, I remember seeing a small, condensed version of myself shrinking down inside my own mind, and for some reason this scared the hell out of me. I just wanted this nightmarish experience to end. Time agonizingly slowed to an almost complete standstill, and it seemed like it was going to be a very long night indeed. "My name is David Jay Brown. I live at 16 Lee Way, Somerville, New Jersey. My name is David Jay Brown . . ."

Then, suddenly, it struck me with the force of a revelation—*Hey, some people actually enjoy this kind of experience!* I became curious about what was happening to me. What could people possibly enjoy about having their minds dissolve? Everything was so intensified. My body was trembling with hypersensitivity, everything was rippling and vibrating, and I was really scared. *Music,* I thought; that seemed worth trying. My mom and brother were asleep in neighboring rooms, so I wrapped a pair of overstuffed stereo headphones around my head and put on an album by the Electric Light Orchestra called *A New World Record.* The first song was called "Livin' Thing."

Within moments I was transported into a state of ecstasy. The music took on incredible depth and dimension audibly, emotionally, and visually, and every note carried me higher and higher into heavenly bliss. I savored the boundless music on my headphones until sunrise, and then at dawn went outside and sat in a lawn chair in my backyard. I looked up at the sky and watched the clouds as everchanging, three-dimensional imagery emerged from them. I stared in pure astonishment at the shifting cartoon and mythiclike images in the sky, as every philosophical or spiritual question that I ever had about God, consciousness, the soul, and reincarnation seemed to be answered immediately in my mind. The answers simply formed in my mind as the questions arose—leaping into my awareness one after another. By the time the sun had risen I knew that I stumbled upon something really big and that my life would be forever changed.

STAYING ONLINE

The eloquent British philosopher Alan Watts is noted for having said that when one gets the message, then one should "hang up the phone," meaning that after one has received the spiritual revelations and mystical insights from a psychedelic experience, there is no need to continue taking the drug. However, I think there is far more than a single message to be gleaned from one's psychedelic experiences, and when you actually have Divine Intelligence on the line, don't you think it might be a bit rude to just hang up? I generally try to keep her talking for as long as I possibly can. Not to mention the fact that human beings have a notorious tendency to forget what they learn, unless it is drilled into them over and over.

It's now been more than thirty-four years since my first acid trip, and I've taken the illegal sacrament well over a thousand times. There's hardly a psychedelic substance listed on the encyclopedic website Erowid that I haven't tried at some point in my career. (I love Erowid! I think that one can effectively argue that Erowid—the largest drug resource on the Internet—has helped to save more lives than any other educational resource in human history.) Additionally, with the exception of only several weeklong or monthlong breaks, I've used cannabis almost every day since I was around fourteen.

At the very least I've been using psychedelic drugs several times a year since that first magical night in 1977, often much more frequently, so it's really impossible for me at this point in my life to even imagine how differently my mind would have developed had I not bathed it in a continuous sea of psychedelic potions since I was a teenager. But it's self-evident that my experimentation with these substances dramatically affected the course of my life and the development of my mind.

Overall, though, I would say that the effects of psychedelics on my life have been overwhelmingly positive. I once debated medical advice "expert" Dr. Drew Pinsky on the popular radio show *Loveline,* which is broadcast on KROQ in Los Angeles. He had been saying repeatedly on the show that LSD caused brain damage, and I knew that this wasn't true. So I told him that there wasn't any scientific evidence to support this notion and that he was spreading misinformation.

To support his frightening claims, Dr. Drew said that while working in psychiatric wards he had witnessed many LSD users who continued to see "trails," blurry tracers following moving objects, long after the acid wore off. It occurred to me that because Dr. Drew was working with the sickest members of our population he tended to pathologize whatever he saw that didn't fit into the conventional psychological mold. In other words, he wasn't working with the best and the brightest LSD users, so he didn't see all the positive and creative changes that I've witnessed.

So I said that I didn't think that this was because of brain damage but rather because of a valid shift in the perception of reality. I've been seeing trails swirling behind everything that moves since I was sixteen, and this seems more like a sense of time dilation to me than brain damage. In fact, on one of the first occasions that I tripped I vividly remembered having seen trails long before, when I was much younger. I saw trails as an infant, before I could talk, and the world seemed to become less and less fluid and more and more solid with time as I grew up.

Psychedelics came into my life just as the magic and innocence of my childhood was leaving. They helped to reconnect me to that magic again, but in a powerful new way, which seemed to jump-start a prewired sequence of developmental phases into action. I think that there actually is something to the notion that marijuana is a gateway drug, but not in the way that most antidrug crusaders would have you believe. There's no scientific or sociological evidence that using cannabis leads to using harder drugs like heroin, cocaine, alcohol, or tobacco. In fact, it appears to be just the opposite, as many of the people who use cannabis tend to become more health-conscious, and many stoners and trippers actually helped to start the health-food industry, as well as many early yoga and fitness centers. Unlike alcohol, cannabis tends to make people more sensitive and aware of their bodies.

However, anyone who has experimented with the classical psychedelics—cannabis (THC), magic mushrooms (psilocybin), peyote (mescaline), or ayahuasca (DMT)—has probably noticed that the effects of these substances have unusual similarities that can seemingly be placed along a continuum. A high dose of cannabis often seems like a low dose of magic mushrooms or LSD. A high dose of LSD or magic mushrooms for many people is like a low dose of DMT or ayahuasca. A low dose of DMT is like a high dose of LSD. So in a sense smoking marijuana prepared me for my LSD experience, and I used the meditation techniques that I had learned prior to using marijuana to help control my marijuana and later my LSD experiences.

Cannabis and LSD opened new gateways to higher states of awareness for me, where the interrelatedness of all things became obvious.

EVERYTHING IS INTERCONNECTED

One of the most valuable lessons that I learned from my psychedelic experiences is that everything is connected to everything else. The vague and gooey revelation from mystical experiences that "all is one" is indeed a profound insight for a mind that has been isolated in the illusion of separateness, and biology and physics absolutely confirm that everything really is interconnected.

All of the boundaries that we routinely see between supposedly separate objects or beings are created and maintained entirely by our conceptual minds—as in nature, every system is simply nestled within a larger system, and everything just flows into everything else. With every breath we take and every move we make, our bodies blend and blur with the environment around us.

Like many other people, the first time that I saw a photograph of the Earth from space, I remember being awestruck by the fact that there were was no clear distinction between the various nations as I had seen on maps of the world in school as a child. I realized on LSD that this was actually true for everything that exists; all and everything is unquestionably, seamlessly interconnected.

It often becomes seemingly obvious to someone under the influence of LSD that our whole planetary biosphere operates as a single organic process, like one organism. James Lovelock's Gaia Hypothesis—which proposes that our oceans and atmosphere are seamlessly regulated by the biosphere itself, so that it maintains the delicate balance of chemicals and conditions that support life on the planet—became an important perspective for me, as well as for many other people who have experimented with psychedelics.

But not everyone whom I interviewed shared this view. When I interviewed Beat poet Allen Ginsberg about the Gaia Hypothesis, he replied:

No, no, no, absolutely not. None of that bullshit! No Gaia hypothesis. No theism need sneak in here. No monotheistic hallucinations needed in this. Not another fascist central authority . . . You've got this one big thing. Who says it's got to be one? Why does everything have to be one? I think there's no such thing as one—only many eyes looking out in all directions. The center is everywhere, not in any one spot. Does it have to be one organism, in the sense of one brain, or one consciousness? The tendency is to sentimentalize this idea into another godhead and to reinaugurate the whole Judeo-Christian-Islamic mind trap.

Nonetheless, many people who use psychedelics report not only is the biosphere capable of intelligent design, but it is a conscious entity that we can dialogue with and learn from. In fact, many people believe that it is absolutely essential that our species understand this if we want to continue to survive and evolve on this planet. I suspect that psychedelic chemicals are messages from the plant world designed to help elevate our environmental awareness and sense of interconnectedness.

Personally, I think that all nationalism is ridiculous. My allegiance is to humanity, to the biosphere, to the Divine Intelligence that organizes the cosmos, not to some silly nation-state government mafia with an army and a flag that thinks it owns the people who live within its artificial borders. Cannabis led me to think this way, and I suspect that this is partially why the giggly healing herb is illegal. It really is quite a challenge to actually believe all their propaganda after one gets sufficiently stoned.

According to researchers at Cardiff University in Britain, above-average intelligence among youth is a risk factor for cannabis use later in life, and Utah criminology professor Gerald Smith identified several warning signs to look for to see if your child is smoking marijuana, such as "excessive preoccupation with social causes, race relations, environmental issues," and so forth.

A lot of people think that the ecology movement sprang largely from the minds of people who had experimented with psychedelics, as many people say that after tripping they can no longer harm the environment without harming themselves. According to mycologist Paul Stamets, psilocybin-containing mushrooms tend to grow in areas where there has been a lot of geological upheaval and activity, like the kind that humans produce. So can it really be a mere coincidence that fungi that tend to make people more ecologically aware also tend to proliferate in areas where humans have radically disrupted the environment?

From an even more transcendent perspective, I just have to wonder about the nature of coincidence in general. Are seemingly profound synchronistic events just unrelated random coincidences that only appear to be ordered and are made meaningful merely by our easily deluded minds? Or is there a designing intelligence lurking behind apparent reality that is somehow creating order? This is one of the most compelling and intriguing questions that I've ever pondered, and it helped to fuel my spiritual and intellectual quest. This also became an important topic of discussion in many of my interviews, and few people had more to say about this fascinating phenomenon than the late author Robert Anton Wilson.

When I asked Wilson what his favorite model for interpreting synchronicity was (as he said that he always had "at least seven models for anything"), he replied:

> Bell's Theorem combined with an idea I got from Barbara Honegger, a parapsychologist . . . She gave me the idea that the right brain is constantly trying to communicate with the left. If you don't listen to what it's trying to say, it gives you more and more vivid dreams— and if you still won't listen, it leads to Freudian slips. If you still don't pay attention, the right brain will get you to the place in space-time where synchronicity will occur. Then the left brain has to pay attention. "Whaaaat!?"

Robert Anton Wilson was one of the smartest and funniest people I ever met, and he came to play a major role in my life.

FIRING THE COSMIC TRIGGER

After turning on to psychedelics I naturally became interested in studying world religions (especially the Eastern philosophies), spirituality, and mysticism, and my interest in science and art was renewed with a passion like never before. I began looking into different psychological and spiritual systems to try to find maps that would help me to understand the unexplored territory of my own mind, and science to validate that what I was seeing was indeed real.

Reading Robert Anton Wilson's book *Cosmic Trigger: Final Secret of the Illuminati* not long after my first LSD trip changed my life again. This is where I first encountered many of the visionaries who would later become the subjects of my interview books, as well as colleagues in my work. As they say in Zen Buddhism, I received the Dharma transmission, so to speak, from Master Wilson. Also of significance, the style in which Wilson's eye-opening book was written inspired the style of the book that you're currently holding in your hands.

What made *Cosmic Trigger* so unique as a literary experiment was how Wilson blended together fascinating and mind-expanding ideas that he was pondering from books that he had read, lively philosophical conversations that he had had with bold and radical thinkers, and ideas from his personal experimentation with psychedelic drugs and other forms of consciousness alteration. These ideas and his experiences resonated deeply with the part of my developing brain that guided the direction of my career choices, my migration patterns, and who I was to become in the context of the world.

Cosmic Trigger is where I first encountered controversial psychologist Timothy Leary's eight-circuit model of the brain and psychiatric researcher John Lilly's radical ideas about programming the brain as though it were a computer. These models became two of the primary maps that I have used to navigate my psychedelic experiences, and Leary introduced me to many other important ideas, which we'll be discussing in more detail later in the book. What's most amazing for me is that later in my life, years after I read Wilson and Leary's work, I was fortunate enough to become good friends with these two incredible gentlemen, and they both played an integral role in my work.

Wilson had an uncanny ability to lead his readers, unsuspectingly, into a state of mind where they are playfully tricked into "aha" experiences that cause them to question their most basic assumptions. His books are the literary equivalent of a psychedelic experience, and they can be every bit as mind-expanding as a couple a good swigs of strong Amazonian jungle juice. Many people, including me, attribute their initial psychological awakening to their reading of his psychoactive books. It was *Cosmic Trigger* that not only allowed me to understand the concept of multiple realities but also inspired me to become a writer when I was a teenager.

I owe a lot to Robert Anton Wilson, or Bob, as he was called by friends. I had completed writing my first book at the age of twenty-six, and I approached him after a lecture that he gave in Santa Cruz, California, to ask him if he would consider writing a promotional blurb for the back cover of the book. He said, "Maybe," and didn't really leave me with the impression that he was too eager to do it. I got the uneasy feeling that young writers bugged him all the time for back-cover blurbs, but he did tell me to have my publisher send him a copy.

So I had my publisher send him a copy of the book. You can hardly imagine my surprise—and total radiant delight—when I discovered that Bob had actually written an eleven-page introduction for the book (*Brainchild,* which was published in 1988 by New Falcon Publications). Words simply cannot describe what a thrilling experience this was for me! In 1989, I moved to Los Angeles, where Bob and his wife, Arlen, were living at the time, and I became good friends with them. I dedicated my book *Virus: The Alien Strain* to Arlen.

I began going to regular weekly gatherings at Bob and Arlen's home, where a small group would read and discuss mind-expanding ideas. We read virtually everything that James Joyce had written, Ezra Pound's *Cantos,* each other's writings, and Bob's books. We watched Orson Welles' films and talked about quantum physics and primate politics. I felt like I was living through a powerful historical event that future generations would surely fantasize about when I got to take part in the *Illuminatus!* trilogy readings and discussions with Bob.

The Illuminatus! trilogy, which Bob coauthored with Robert Shea, is probably Bob's best-known book, and it was the first book of his that I read, at age fifteen. *Illuminatus!* is a densely written, stream-of-consciousness science-fiction novel about political conspiracies that breaks every rule of language and manages to transcend everything that one thinks a book can do. Reading James Joyce's *Ulysses* and Thomas Pynchon's *Gravity's Rainbow* had a similar effect on me years later.

I continued going to weekly gatherings at Bob's home until a few weeks before he died. He remained as sharp and witty as ever right up until the end. I saw Bob around once a week for seventeen years, during which time he played a huge role in my writing career. He was incredibly supportive of my writing. He wrote letters to cheer me up when I was down and even sent me money when I couldn't afford to pay my rent.

I interviewed Bob for my first book of interviews, *Mavericks of the Mind,* in 1989 and again for my third interview collection, *Conversations on the Edge of the Apocalypse,* in 2004. He wrote blurbs for the back covers of my other books as well, and he mentioned me in a few of his books—which always gave me a thrill. Bob often gave me credit in his books for coming up with the abbreviation BS for *belief system,* although I was given this abbreviation by my late friend Allyn Brodsky. But one of the happiest days in my writing career came when Bob actually asked me to write a back-cover blurb for his book *TSOG: The Thing That Ate the Constitution.* Wow—now that blew my mind. I was working on my book *Mavericks of Medicine* while Bob was dying, and I dedicated the book to him.

Bob had an uncanny ability to perceive things that few people notice, and he had an incredible memory. He had an encyclopedic knowledge of many different fields, ranging from literature and psychology to quantum physics and neuroscience. He was unusually creative in his use of language, and he had his own unique style of humor and satire. Despite many serious personal challenges over the years, Bob always maintained a strongly upbeat, optimistic, and cheerful perspective on life, and—regardless of the circumstances—he never failed to make me smile every time I saw him. Everyone who met him agrees; there was something truly magical about Robert Anton Wilson.

CHANGING ONE'S MIND AMONG THE GREATEST MINDS OF OUR TIME

The radical ideas that I picked up from Robert Anton Wilson, as well as from the other extraordinary people whom I began to interview for my books, intermingled with my own ever-changing thoughts while I was high or tripping, and this is how my ideas for more questions developed. I've been extremely fortunate and have been able to interview and spend time with virtually every influential member of the psychedelic community who has lived during my lifetime.

The people whom I choose to interview for my collections are largely the same people whose books I passionately enjoyed reading and whose ideas I liked to think about when I was in the process of melting and expanding my mind. Over time I experienced a kind of organic unfolding process as my own experiences and insights influenced what I was interacting with my interviewees about, and vice versa. This process was greatly enhanced by the development of the Internet, so that I now feel like the writers behind almost every new book I read are easily accessible to me if I have any questions about their work or would like to conduct an interview with any of them.

It seems like we're all part of a single mind, grappling with the same ideas, trying to grasp our place in the universe. Computer philosopher Francis Jeffrey gave me some invaluable advice early in my career. He said that whenever I enjoy reading a book I should contact the author and tell him or her how much I liked it. He said that I would be surprised how many authors would be happy to hear from me. He was right.

One of the most important things I learned about conducting interviews is how important trust is. I learned from media personality Phil Donahue that it's helpful to treat famous people like they're not famous, and ordinary people like they are famous. I've noticed that this helps people to open up and feel comfortable during an interview. I also listen a lot.

Since I began conducting interviews with exceptional thinkers, I've been particularly interested in how psychedelics affect creativity and enhance the imagination. One of the primary goals of my interview books and my work with the Multidisciplinary Association for Psychedelic Studies (MAPS), which we'll be discussing later, has been to document the important role that psychedelics have had in influencing some of the most accomplished and influential people on the planet.

I think it is important for future generations that this valuable information isn't lost because of cultural taboos, misunderstandings, and government repression. Psychedelics have played an invaluable role in the development of numerous scientific discoveries and artistic inspirations, not to mention political revolutions, which I think have helped to change the world for the better.

For example, the biotechnology revolution was largely started by two Nobel Prize biochemists, Francis Crick and Kary Mullis, who both reportedly attributed part of their insights to their use of LSD. Crick, along with James Watson, discovered the double-helix structure of the DNA molecule—the genetic code—and, according to a BBC report, sources close to Crick say that he was regularly using low doses of LSD at the time of the discovery. When I interviewed Mullis—who developed the polymerase chain reaction (PCR), which revolutionized the study of genetics and made genetic engineering possible—he told me, "I think I might have been stupid in some respects, if it weren't for my psychedelic experiences." Steve Jobs, one of the cofounders of Apple, told *New York Times* reporter John Markoff that his LSD experiences were among "the two or three most important experiences" of his life.

In the sixties and seventies the use of psychedelics by creative people in the music industry helped to spawn technologies that combined new forms of music with laser light shows, and magic mushroom–munching filmmakers were inspired to develop new cinematic techniques that used special effects to mimic the perceptual effects of hallucinogens. For example, Stanley Kubrick, who directed *2001: A Space Odyssey,* was turned on to LSD by Los Angeles psychiatrist Oscar Janiger when the drug was still legal.

These days it's hard to even see a television commercial that doesn't seem to be influenced by psychedelics. "Taste the rainbow," proclaims a Skittles commercial. The truth is, there is hardly an area of human culture—art, science, medicine, politics, music, philosophy, and spirituality—that psychedelics haven't immensely impacted. However, this impact is often demonized, trivialized, or overlooked by the dominant ruling-class culture.

I've asked many dozens of accomplished visionaries about how their psychedelic experiences have affected their creativity and have gotten some pretty fascinating responses over the years. A number of the people I interviewed even opened up with me, publicly for the first time, about their use of psychedelics, such as neuroscientist Candace Pert, spiritual teacher Deepak Chopra, NASA astronaut Edgar Mitchell, and the late psychiatric researcher John Mack. We'll be discussing this in more detail later in the book.

My psychedelic-inspired interests and the people whom I've interviewed have led me through an intellectual and mystical carnival ride where the unexpected continuously revealed itself to me, and this adventure became the basis for this book. Some of the fascinating ideas that we'll be exploring in this volume include speculations about the nature of consciousness, intelligence and creativity, unexplained phenomena in science, and the relationship between science and spirituality.

We'll be examining an intriguing array of mind-boggling questions that challenge our limited views of reality: What kind of an effect do psychedelics have on creativity and the imagination? What happens to consciousness after death? Is time travel possible? Have people really made contact with extraterrestrials, the spirit world, or the dead? Will the human species survive, or are we doomed to extinction? How can we become more ecologically aware as a species and live in a more sustainable way with our biosphere?

If we do survive, how will the human species evolve in the future? Is consciousness or psychic phenomena scientifically measurable? What causes all of the weird, unexplained phenomena in the world, like crop circles and alien abductions? Is the term *God* truly meaningful, and, if so, what does it mean exactly? What do genetic modification, advanced robotics, artificial intelligence, and nanotechnology hold in store for us? How can we become smarter and live longer, happier lives?

These questions (and others), which I am still exploring today, came to me on my psychedelic experiences, and they provided the inspiration for my many interviews and gave me a lot to contemplate on my additional psychedelic journeys.

1

Head West and Get High, Young Man

After I completed my master's degree in neuroscience at New York University in 1986, I drove across country to California, the place that I love more than anywhere else on Earth. After working in a cramped neuroscience lab for two years in New York City, doing electrical brain-stimulation research on rats, I was ready to let my mind and spirit burst free. During my beautiful, awe-inspiring, cannabis-fueled drive across the country, the entire outline for my first book, the science-fiction novel *Brainchild,* bubbled up effortlessly in my head. I had to keep pulling over to the side of the road while I was driving to write down my continuous flow of ever-multiplying ideas.

Heading west was important to me, and I've lived in California for most of my adult life. I learned from Leary and Wilson that for thousands of years the most experimentally minded and culturally innovative people have been steadily migrating in a westward pattern around the planet. I read Leary's essay "Spinning Up the Genetic Highway" (in his book *The Intelligence Agents*) when I was tripping on blotter acid during a break from college at the age of eighteen, and I realized that I needed to move to California as soon as possible if I wanted to find other people who thought like I did. Someone once asked Leary, "What do you do after you turn on?" Leary replied, "Find the others."

I've always been amazed by how quickly I can tell whether a person whom I've just met has ever done psychedelics at some point in his life. I estimate that I can judge this with around 95 percent accuracy after just a few minutes of talking with the person. I've met other people who tell me that they can do this too, and it appears to be an ability that is genetically wired into our species. It seems that people who have used psychedelics are able to recognize signals from other people who also have, and these signals remain invisible to people who have never had a psychedelic experience.

When someone is faking psychedelic knowledge it is usually easy to spot, and it's why narcotics officers often look silly to stoners and trippers. There's also something in particular that I can't quite put my finger on about the way that someone who has had a powerful psychedelic experience will look me in the eyes, which gives me an instant sense of kinship. And the faces of people who have tripped seem more fluid, more animated, and more emotionally expressive to me. Again, this is pretty difficult to fake, and my intuitions have largely been confirmed over the years, but not always.

I mentioned this ability that psychedelic users have to recognize one another to my friend Danielle Bohmer, and she said, "It's true. You can just tell. It reminds me of the Frank Zappa line, 'I will have a psychedelic gleam in my eye at all times.'" I found her response to be especially interesting, because Frank Zappa is actually one of the very few people who totally fooled me. After listening to his wonderfully fantastic, supertrippy music, I was very surprised to discover that he never tripped on psychedelics. Some people just seem to have naturally psychedelic brains.

However, I can also usually sense a psychedelic influence when examining an artistic creation—in a book, painting, sculpture, performance, film, or musical composition—and I noticed as a teenager that lots of psychedelic cultural signals were coming from California.

Westward migration made sense to me while I was tripping, because I realized that migrating west means that you're moving against the spin of the planet, which spins from east to west. From an extraterrestrial vantage point (i.e., high off the planet) moving west can be seen as a climb upward over time, as though humans for thousands of years have been faithfully ascending a giant mountain that stretches from India to Hawaii.

If one studies the history of human civilizations, it seems that those areas of the world where people have been the most culturally experimental and technologically innovative have steadily moved west since the beginning of the first developed countries that exist to this day.

The oldest surviving nations on the planet can be found in the East, and those places where great cultural advancements have taken place seem to light up in a westward (i.e., upwardly) directional sequence, beginning in India and China, expanding into the Middle East, and winding into eastern Europe, then into western Europe and Great Britain, to the east coast of America, and finally to the west coast of America, where California and Hawaii represent the current peaks of this global migration process.

When one travels eastward from California, one encounters societies that have increasingly older and older histories, less and less tolerance for individual differences, more and more suspicion about anything new or different, and greater and greater respect for and attachment to authority and tradition. Traveling west from China, one sees this pattern going in reverse, until one reaches California and Hawaii, where there is considerable lifestyle and cultural experimentation and tolerance for individual differences. I agree with Wilson and Leary that traveling eastward takes you into the past, and moving westward carries you into the future. The planetary time zones on Earth should not be separated by hours, Leary said, but rather by centuries.

These westward migration patterns made sense to me in the larger context of understanding that there was an evolutionary momentum behind human progress, moving it ever upward, and I realized that there was a long history indeed behind getting high. Our early ancestors climbed up out of the ocean on to dry land. Then they grew taller, rose onto their hind legs, and began climbing into the trees. Some animals took off into the air and learned to fly; we eventually learned to do so as well with our technology.

The locus of consciousness in every animal species is always located near the top of its head—as close to the Heavens as physiologically possible, which has the highest perceptual vantage point. When I've done LSD or psilocybin I often felt like the locus of my consciousness shifted from the center of my head to a point that is actually a few inches above my head. It is no accident, I realized, that people refer to cannabis intoxication as a high. Consciousness has been literally evolving higher and higher for eons; the brains of animals evolved into higher and higher positions of physical elevation throughout our evolution, and the cannabis plant seemed to be hitching a ride on this trend. Throughout evolution consciousness has been rising upward, against the force of gravity, toward the stars.

After considering all of this one just has to ask: Why was California primarily settled from Europe and not Asia? Where were all the great Asian explorers in history? Why did the world explorers who settled the Americas come primarily from western Europe and not eastern Asia? Why is California so psychedelic, so tolerant and open-minded, and so culturally experimental compared to the rest of the world? The answers to these questions, I suspect, reside in our understanding of planetary spin. We evolved by moving upward, by getting high, by moving against the spin of the Earth.

PSYCHEDELICS, EVOLUTION, AND SENSORY DEPRIVATION TANKS

Evolution has been moving consciousness higher and higher for billions of years, and it seems that there is currently no other direction to go than up. It appears that the inevitable next step in this evolutionary process involves our species' migration off the planet's surface and into space. I often wonder if we are being prepared by cannabis and psychedelics for life in zero gravity, where we can frolic gravity-free in high-orbiting space colonies within self-contained biospheres. Or, perhaps, for reaching into the depths of outer space, to encounter new forms of intelligent life or into higher dimensions of reality. In this context I often wonder why science-fiction space fantasies are so popular among trippers and stoners.

When I interviewed NASA astronaut Edgar Mitchell, the sixth man to walk on the moon, he told me that his mystical experiences in zero gravity were similar to his experiences with LSD. When I asked Mitchell to describe what his mystical experience in space was like, he replied:

> I suddenly realized that the molecules of my body, the molecules of the spacecraft, and those of my partners, had been prototyped in some ancient generation of stars. And, okay, that was nice intellectual knowledge, but all of a sudden it hit me at the gut, and—wow—those are my molecules. It became personal. I could see the stars, see the separateness of things, but felt an inner connectedness of everything. It was personal. It was wild. It was ecstatic.

Sharing a few beers with an open-minded space-shuttle astronaut one night in New York City after an L-5 meeting, he confided in me that all astronauts get high and euphoric after a few days in zero gravity, but very few speak about this.

According to NASA psychologist Steve Groff, many astronauts were given psychedelic drugs by NASA—LSD and a top-secret drug, which was likely JB-118, JB-318, or a ketamine analog—to prepare them for the weightlessness of space and the disorientation that may come from a lack familiar external cues.

My own experiences floating in the sensory-deprivation tanks (that my late friend John Lilly designed) convinced me that just removing the physical restriction of gravity from the body can free the mind and allow it to soar through the higher spheres. Floating in a sensory-deprivation tank can produce an experience very similar to that of psychedelic drugs or a lucid dream. (I spent around a year doing ketamine regularly with John Lilly, and sometimes alone in his isolation tank, at his estate high in the Malibu mountains. I will be discussing this more later in the book.)

Every weekend for four years during the early 1980s, while I was studying psychobiology at USC in Los Angeles, I worked at an isolation tank, biofeedback, entrainment brain machine center called the Altered States Relaxation Center in West Hollywood. I gave orientations to dozens of people about how to use the tanks, and I logged many hours in them after closing on weekend nights, when I had the place all to myself. I experimented with various psychedelic drugs in the tanks and had some truly extraordinary experiences. For example, one night while tripping on magic mushrooms in the tank, and after becoming "unstuck in time," I got out to go the bathroom. Seeing myself in the mirror with huge, unnaturally bulging alien eyes convinced me that I had permanently altered my DNA and I was now a new species. I still wonder if this is true.

A lot of interesting people came to the Altered States Relaxation Center. One afternoon I gave an orientation to a beautiful young woman and her partner. I felt particularly charismatic and confident that day for some reason, and I enjoyed talking with the friendly couple a lot. After they were behind closed doors in their private room, ready to immerse themselves in the tanks, and I was sitting at the desk, the co-owner of the establishment approached me and said, "Do you know who that woman was that you gave an orientation to?" I had no idea, but I thought that she was really cute and I had a crush on her. "That was Carrie Fisher. You know, Princess Leia from *Star Wars*?" he said. Then it dawned on me—yes, of course that's why she looked familiar.

Around ten minutes later, while I was alone in the office, Carrie came walking out of the private tank and shower room all alone, wrapped in nothing but a small towel around her beautiful body. She stood by a small table just a few feet away and smiled. We were alone in the room together, and now that I knew who she was, all my confidence and charisma completely vanished and I was just blinking at her, speechless and starstruck. She looked radiantly sexy, and I was completely tongue-tied.

Carrie then said that she wanted to pay me for the session. I said that this wasn't necessary until the end of the session, but she insisted that she wanted to pay now. Then she sat down at the table across from me. We sat there together in complete silence as she slowly wrote out a check, close enough that I could smell how good she smelled, but I was just too nervous to say a word. Our hands touched momentarily when she handed me the check, and a shiver of electricity traveled up my arm. I anxiously considered asking her to have lunch with me sometime as I watched the sensuous movements of her naked shoulders, but she went back into the tank room before I said anything, likely puzzled—or maybe not—by the dramatic change in my personality.

I hadn't been that starstruck since I coincidentally got into the elevator at the USC Annenberg School for Communication building with the legendary designer R. Buckminster Fuller and his family. Bucky, as he was called, started introducing me to his family in the elevator, and I didn't know what else to say besides "Nice to meet you." Years later I asked Bucky to write something in my private journal, on the first page, under the title "Amazing Days." Bucky wrote, *To David, All days are amazing.* I also asked the late comedy science-fiction writer Douglas Adams to do the same thing. Adams wrote simply, *Don't Panic!*

In any case, Carrie went back into the isolation tank room, and afterward, with others, we spoke for around a half hour about her experience in the tank. We spoke for a bit about John Lilly's work, and she told me that she would be terrified to ever do psychedelics in the tank. To this day I have a very warm spot in my heart for Carrie Fisher and am a huge fan of the *Star Wars* films in which she starred.

The *Star Wars* films have an archetypal or mythic quality to them, where past and future seem to merge. Myths and archetypes are universal in the human species, and they appear to be genetically wired into us. Psychedelics can activate a state of consciousness that seems to put us in touch with the source of these archetypal patterns, an illuminated superintelligence shining inside our DNA molecules.

DEVELOPING GENETIC AWARENESS

It's not far-fetched to suspect that psychedelics activate a kind of genetic awareness, a state of consciousness that sees the world from an evolutionary perspective. We know, for example, that lower psychedelic doses of the dissociative anesthetic ketamine will turn on certain genes that a full anesthetic dose won't. Psychedelic doses can induce DNA to produce the c-Fos protein, among others, and the knockout doses of ketamine do not. In other words, it seems that our DNA recognizes when we're tripping.

Recent genetic research suggests that much of the DNA molecule that was thought to be unnecessary "junk" (rather than mystery DNA, as anthropologist Jeremy Narby pointed out in his book *The Cosmic Serpent: DNA and the Origins of Knowledge*) may actually contain a wealth of valuable information. Some of this "junk" may contain past-life memories as previous organisms and maybe even anticipated possibilities or designs for the future, such as sensual intelligence, psychic abilities, DNA self-awareness, and access to hidden dimensions of the mind, which I'll discuss more later. As our study of gene activation by drugs becomes more sophisticated, "junk DNA" may play a vital role in future research that explores new brain states and alterations in consciousness.

There is a drawing by artist Peter Von Sholly in Timothy Leary's book *The Game of Life* that made a deep impression on me when I was tripping on acid one night as a teenager in my New Jersey bedroom. Von Sholly's drawing was meant to illustrate a stage of psychological or neurological development that Leary termed "neurogenetic awareness." This roughly corresponded to what the late psychologist Carl Jung called the "collective unconsciousness," or what psychiatric researcher Stanislav Grof refers to as "phylogenetic awareness."

On high doses of psychedelics it is common for people to see the biosphere, the world, the evolutionary process, human history, and the future from a genetic perspective, from the point of view of a DNA molecule—the molecular intelligence residing inside the nucleus of every living cell. DNA directs the show of life on this planet, and I'm fairly convinced that it does so consciously, intelligently, and compassionately, with a higher purpose in mind. As a voice once told pharmacologist Dennis McKenna when he was tripping on ayahuasca, "You monkeys only think you're running the show."

Von Sholly's illustration replaces God and Adam in Michelangelo's famous painting of God creating Adam with a winged, male insectoid-humanoid creature joining hands with a petal-flowering, female botanical-humanoid creature. I saw in this drawing a new understanding of interspecies symbiosis that I suspect lies in our future. This made me wonder about that erotic feeling I get whenever I watch a field of flowers intermingle with honeybees, and it inspired a new understanding of why we often refer to sexuality as the birds and the bees. Leary said that this phrase was really meant to be the *blooms and the bees,* which makes a lot more sense when you think about it.

It suddenly hit me with the force of a revelation that when bees are buzzing around from flower to flower on a sunny summer day collecting pollen to make honey, they're not only fertilizing the flowers, they're also making love to them. It's a form of interspecies symbiosis that vividly expresses the sexuality of nature.

It occurred to me that because of their tiny size insects have progressed through what appears to be a universal evolutionary sequence more quickly than we have, and winged social insects could be useful, it seems, to help us forecast aspects of our evolutionary future as flying post-terrestrial beings who form symbiotic sexual unions with flowering plants—as they're physically ahead of us on the evolutionary sequence. We appear to be at a level similar to those of terrestrial social insects, like ants or termites, on our way to becoming something like mammalian bees and cyborg butterflies.

Leary attempted to show that life on Earth evolves in the same way that many other dynamic processes in the universe develop, according to the law of octaves and the periodic table of elements, and that we can surmise that this pattern is likely to occur all over the universe wherever life evolves. The law of octaves shows that what we perceive as the rainbow, the visible color spectrum, or the range of musical notes is the key to understanding how many processes in the universe progress—from the life cycles of stars, to the colors that a wound goes through when it heals, to human development and the evolution of different species.

Only a small number of animal species are bound to the surface of the ground for life; most animals live their adult lives primarily in the ocean or the air. It makes sense then, if life has any kind of teleological direction, that land animals would just be a transitional phase in the evolutionary process, and human beings—from this vantage point—are merely a larval form of what's to come. This is probably why so many people dream of flying; it may be preprogrammed for us to yearn for a way to master gravity, and this may be what cannabis and psychedelic mind states are preparing us for. This may also help to explain our species' fascination with the artistic renderings of angels and fairies, as these winged beings may be precognitive flashes of ourselves in the future.

Terence McKenna, the late ethnobotanist whom I interviewed at the start of my career and who was another influential figure in my life, proposed that magic mushrooms provided the stimulus that awakened the evolutionary potential in early humans to develop language. McKenna postulated that magic mushrooms might be an alien species from outer space and that they had a significant and catalytic effect on our evolution.

My own experiences with psilocybin mushrooms seemed to confirm, with a great deal of certainty, that residing within the mushroom there is indeed an intelligent entity with which one can dialogue, if one is brave enough to consume the flesh of the fungi in significant enough quantities. (McKenna's recipe for a dialogue with the mushroom spirit was five dried grams of *Psilocybe cubensis* in silent darkness.) If this dialogue is an illusion, it sure is an extremely convincing one, as it appears that a growing number of people are merging their consciousness with the ancient mushroom mind. This makes me wonder if we aren't beginning, as a species, to form a symbiotic union with intelligent fungi and plants. We'll be talking more about McKenna's ideas later in the book.

When I was taking some graduate school courses at the University of California, Santa Cruz in 1984 my interest in evolution and psychology led to intimate encounters with the politically controversial science of sociobiology—which is about how behaviors can be genetically encoded and evolve through the process of natural selection. I studied with acclaimed evolutionary biologist Robert Trivers at UC Santa Cruz during the mid-1980s and often debated my ideas with him. He didn't seem to be terribly impressed by the Gaia Hypothesis or the idea of teleology operating in nature, but he did agree to participate in a debate that Rebecca Novick and I were planning on McKenna's theory of how human evolution had been influenced by psilocybin mushrooms in the diet of our early ancestors. Unfortunately it never took place, but the interview Rebecca and I did with Trivers can be found in our book *Mavericks of the Mind,* alongside our interview with McKenna.

Penn State professor Richard Doyle wrote a fascinating book on sex, plants, and the evolution of the noosphere called *Darwin's Pharmacy,* and it sheds some interesting light on the notion that humans are unwittingly participating in a partnership with psychedelic plants. In science-fiction writer Norman Spinrad's book *Child of Fortune,* one of my favorite books of all time, there is a marvelous section where the protagonist is traveling through the Bloomenvelt forest, a place in which flowering plants form symbiotic relationships with human beings. Humans are lured in to this seductive garden by plants that produce intoxicating olfactory drugs and delicious, impossible-to-resist fruits that turn humans into mindlessly copulating pollinators for the plants. Both of these books seem to me like communications from a neurogenetic state of consciousness.

In any case, largely because of my psychedelic experiences I began to accept the teleological notion that our evolution has a built-in design to it, a design that we could learn to access, decode, and eventually override with psychedelics and advanced biotechnology. The states of mind that cannabis and psychedelics activate appear to be lying dormant as natural states in all human beings. Similar states of consciousness could be caused by means other than drugs or plants—such as meditation, sensory deprivation, body/mind control exercises, fasting, and near-death shock—and there seems to be a recognizable developmental sequence that people will progress through once these dormant brain centers have been awakened. Leary, Wilson, and numerous others have tried to map out and model this developmental sequence.

I suspect that all life on this planet is akin to a tree growing from a seed; the design was encoded from the start. The urge to get high is instinctive; it is genetically wired into us from birth. The desire to recreationally ingest psychoactive drugs is deeply rooted in our biological nature. The hunger to get high is as natural as the desire to eat, sleep, and procreate. Young children have an instinctive drive to change their ordinary state of awareness, as evidenced by the delight that they take in spinning around and around in circles to produce a state of dizziness. According to UCLA psychopharmacologist Ron Siegel, every human culture and every animal species makes use of certain plants for their psychoactive properties. In fact, Siegel believes that "the desire for intoxication is actually a fourth drive, as unstoppable as hunger, thirst, and sex."

WHY ARE PSYCHEDELIC DRUGS ILLEGAL?

There are a number of important reasons why world governments are so genuinely frightened of psychedelic substances and there is a strong cultural taboo around them. Scientific evidence supports the fact that the draconian prohibition currently being practiced is most definitely not because of the danger of physical or psychological harm, especially because these substances are known to be so physically safe and so many medical benefits are now being discovered for them. Not to mention the fact that nowhere in the U.S. Constitution does it say that the government is allowed to "protect us" from the consequences of our own free and informed choices that don't harm others.

Hidden under the guise of protecting people from a nonexistent health menace, the governments' true agenda—conscious or not—appears to be to suppress people from activating states of consciousness that allow them to transcend cultural value systems, to think for themselves, and to question the authority of their culture's values. Psychedelics dissolve personal and conceptual boundaries. They put one in touch with something deeper than culture, a primordial genetic awareness, and the flaws of an antiquated culture, and the ways that it can be improved become obvious. It's very hard for someone who has tasted the cultural transcendence that psychedelics offer to ever fall for the deceptive manipulations of the corporate-controlled media, and there are unquestionably government officials who are aware of this.

The late ethnobotanist Terence McKenna said:

> Psychedelics are illegal not because a loving government is concerned that you might jump out of a third story window. Psychedelics are illegal because they dissolve opinion structure and culturally-laid-down models of behavior and information processing. They open you up to the possibility that everything you know is wrong.

However, what seems to infuriate people who have never done psychedelics most of all is that people who have done psychedelics often find those who have never tripped to be extremely funny. Stoners and trippers commonly laugh at the unquestioned rituals of conventional, materialistic, consumer society, and they tend to mock straight society's serious, consumer-driven attitudes toward money, greed, and power. I suspect that this humorous attitude toward conventional customs is, again, a genetically wired response from activating our higher brain circuits, although it sure can upset some people. But this may be because the controversy and attention is actually necessary to spread the word about cannabis and psychedelics around the globe. It may be that cannabis and psychedelics are illegal because genetic intelligence recognizes that this is simply the best way to inform people about them. Nonetheless, as Timothy Leary once said, "LSD can cause psychotic reactions in people who haven't taken it."

MY ENCOUNTER WITH HOMELAND SECURITY

My late friend and the brilliant neuroscientist John C. Lilly once warned me that if we start to evolve too quickly the evolutionary police might come after us for exceeding the evolutionary speed limit on this planet. I think that John's caution was well founded, as the long and notorious legal troubles of our mutual friend Timothy Leary clearly demonstrate.

While I'm sure that I couldn't possibly pose much political threat to anyone, I've been honest and publicly outspoken about the benefits that I've gained from psychedelics for more than thirty-five years, and this hasn't always attracted the most positive attention. In July of 2009 I received a visit from the U.S. Department of Homeland Security. They were following up on an anonymous letter they had received from someone stating that I was a dangerous cult leader brainwashing young women with mind-altering drugs with the goal of training them to assassinate the president.

I found a notification from the ominous government department hanging on my door after receiving a rather frantic phone call from a friend who was interning at the Multidisciplinary Association for Psychedelic Studies (MAPS) office that summer. She told me that there were government agents at the office that day asking some of the employees at MAPS detailed questions about me. They asked about a half-dozen people there and elsewhere about me and whether I was running a dangerous cult.

Of course I've never led any such cult and have always been a pacifist, so at first it all seemed too ridiculous to take seriously, and I found the situation rather amusing. Then I spoke with a trusted attorney at the ACLU about it. He told me to take the situation seriously because of how outspoken I've been about the benefits of psychedelic drugs, and he advised me not to talk to any government officials without having my attorney present. I was glad that I took his advice and let my attorney handle the matter. Once my attorney called the Department of Homeland Security they were no longer interested in questioning me.

Apparently the jealous ex-boyfriend of a woman I was spending time with wrote a letter to the FBI, and although everything in it was entirely fabricated, my attorney warned me that government agents could use this as an opportunity to get me to talk about my use of illegal psychedelic drugs. I've saved them a lot of work by simply writing this book. Robert Anton Wilson used to forward every one of his e-mail correspondences to National Security Advisor John Poindexter, who created the Information Awareness Office to spy on Americans while George W. Bush was president in order to save Poindexter the trouble of having to obtain his e-mails by spying.

Because I rarely use psychedelics anymore I didn't think I had anything to worry about, but I'm glad that I followed my attorney's advice. I learned that one never has to talk to a government agent without having an attorney present to represent him or her. Speaking only with an attorney present is not a sign of guilt but rather of intelligence. "It's what any person of means would do," my attorney told me.

Despite being pretty spooked at times like this, I've realized that being fortunate enough to experience the glorious transcendental magic of psychedelics is a call to spiritual duty. As the late physicist Albert Einstein once said, "Those who have the privilege to know, have the duty to act." Marvel comic book writer Stan Lee echoed this by saying, "With great power comes great responsibility."

If we learn how to improve our lives with psychedelics I think it's our responsibility, our sacred duty, to share what we've learned with the rest of the world. Our planet is in a serious crisis right now, and we really need everyone's help. I doubt that the great goddess of psychedelia revealed all of her sacred wisdom to us just to make our personal lives better. I think that we must go out and share what we've learned with others.

Let us not forget that our primary goal right now is to help elevate awareness on this planet enough to keep our species from going extinct and to make it to the next evolutionary stage. Everyone is needed to make this happen! So if you're awake and you're not working to help wake up others, then watch out. The Chinese military or the American corporations may come and force you to share your wisdom with the world—just look at what happened to Tibet and the Amazonian rain forest. It's doubtful that the world would be celebrating the wisdom of the Dalai Lama, or that ayahuasca religions would be popping up like mushrooms around the globe, had it not been for the Chinese invasion of Tibet or the corporate exploitation of the Amazon. The biosphere needs our help now.

People with rigid minds who have a lot invested in the old power structures will desperately cling to preserving the old values and reject anything that threatens their power until new, younger, and more open-minded people come along to replace them. I suspect that the tipping point is almost here.

SOLVING THE WORLD'S PROBLEMS WITH SHAMANIC VISION

I think that it's natural for humans to consume psychoactive plants that alter their neurochemistry as a way of learning more about themselves and the world, and this is why I think that America's War on Drugs is really a war on human nature. (R. A. Wilson was always fond of calling it, more accurately, the War on Some Drugs.) The social and political agendas of the developed countries in this world appear to be completely out of touch with the environmental dangers that we're currently facing and which threaten our very existence as a species. But I think many of the world's most pressing problems can be traced to three human practices that people rarely question: male circumcision, alarm clocks, and watching the evening news on television.

To have one's most sensitive organ sliced open and torn apart without anesthetic, as a newborn, has been shown to create lasting trauma in the brain in the area of the amygdala, which is responsible for fear and aggression. For most men I suspect that it lasts a lifetime. Cultural comparison studies have shown that societies that circumcise their male newborns tend to be more violent and aggressive than societies that don't. For example, in two of the most violent and aggressive places in the world—America and the Middle East—it is routine for many male newborns to be circumcised.

Circumcision turns an unusually sensitive inner organ into a calloused, insensitive outer organ and emotionally scars the owner for life. It destroys all of the fine-touch nerve endings in the head of the penis. I think that this barbaric practice—which probably had some benefit to warring tribes—is a huge contribution to all of the unrestrained fear and aggression in the world. This, I suspect, is further heightened by the global prohibition of cannabis, which appears to temper male aggression.

Male circumcision creates a negative neurological imprint of the world, telling us that the world is not a safe place and we should either fear it or fight against it. Imprinting is a biological phenomenon that was discovered by ethologist Konrad Lorenz when he found out that newborn ducks would follow him around like a mama duck if he was the very first thing they saw upon hatching. This period of imprint vulnerability is brief, and the effects can last a lifetime. Few people have applied imprint theory to human psychology, but Leary and Wilson theorize that psychedelic drugs suspend cultural imprints and allow us to more carefully and consciously choose new ones.

Alarm clocks disrupt natural sleep cycles, which has numerous negative effects on mood, intelligence, and health. I think it's been overlooked by most people how much the practice of waking up to an alarm clock every day is creating anxiety, depression, and confusion in their lives. This is, of course, reinforced by the television evening news, which delivers all of the most horrible and gruesome things that happened on the planet that day into your living room, reinforcing the notion that the world is a dangerous and scary place that we need protection from—except when it's time for the commercials, when the world becomes a happy place if you simply purchase largely useless products.

Certainly solving all the environmental, political, and social problems in the world is a whole lot more complicated than changing these three simple things, but I think that addressing these problems might be a good place to start. How to solve our wayward world's most pressing problems became an important theme for many of my interviews, which we'll explore later in this book.

EVERYONE IS OMNIPOTENT AND ALL POWERFUL

Another one of the valuable lessons that I learned from tripping was that I had the power to make anything happen as long as I executed the correct sequence of behaviors or actions and really believed in myself. This insight came from putting together two obvious truths.

First, take a look around you right now. You'll see that, with the exception of the natural world, everything that exists around you in the urban world—every single constructed object inside of every building—first existed inside of the mind of a human being. All that exists in our self-created world sprang out of someone's imagination. And truth number two: the one and only domain where you rule supreme is your own mind. When you couple these two obvious truths you realize that you have enormous power if you *just put your mind to it*.

This is also why no one is ever totally helpless. No matter what sort of circumstances people find themselves in, at the very least everyone always has the ability to control how they react to those circumstances. The late Austrian psychiatrist Viktor Frankl, author of *Man's Search for Meaning,* demonstrated that this was possible even under the most horrific of circumstances, such as when he was a prisoner in a Nazi concentration camp. He said, "Between stimulus and response there is a space. In that space is our power to choose our response. In our response lies our growth and our freedom." The greatest truth of all is that ultimately no one can completely control our minds but ourselves.

Sometimes just putting two ideas together that I already knew but hadn't quite realized how they enhanced one another's meaning would allow me to communicate the essence of a profound psychedelic revelation. For example, I also realized that when on psychedelics, who we identify with as our true selves is most definitely not our physical bodies, and this is why, in speech, we instinctively refer to our bodies as something separate from ourselves, as something that we own or inhabit.

I've always wondered why even fundamentalist materialists use the expressions *my body* instead of *I am a body,* and if this means that people generally feel like they are a ghostly field of consciousness inhabiting a physical body, like a hand inside of a glove. I'm perplexed by people who think that consciousness is just an epiphenomenon of the brain but then use the expression *my brain.* People even use the expression *my soul,* which is even harder for me to understand, unless one has the perspective of an oversoul, which, according to New England transcendentalism, is a spiritual essence that all souls in the universe participate in and which therefore transcends individual consciousness. Whose soul are people talking about it? If people aren't their bodies, minds, or souls, I'm not really sure what they are.

But we can't simply be just our physical bodies. Every single atom in our bodies is completely replaced every few years, and physically we are merely the pattern that endures. Whatever we ultimately are, it seems that the core of our being is more like an organizing field than a physical form, which itself is nestled nonlocally within ever higher and higher organizing fields. When this understanding is coupled with the evidence of field effects in microbiology, the insight deepens. If you stick a microneedle into the nucleus of a cell and swish the DNA apart, it will reorganize its original structure by largely mysterious means, like iron filings around a magnet.

We know that some *E. coli* bacteria don't mutate randomly. Rather, they mutate in a way that corresponds to environmental pressures, so their mutations are more likely to adapt to the new environment than purely random mutations would. I discussed with biochemist Kary Mullis the implications of this research as possibly shedding some light on whether there is a form of intelligence that plays a teleological role in evolution. He said that although he was aware of this study he did not think that it implied any type intelligence in evolution. He said he thought this nonrandomly mutating process that seemed intelligent had itself simply evolved purely randomly through a process of natural selection. While this may be possible, I'm not sure I agree, mostly because of my sense of intuition. I think these interesting results may provide evidence that nature is intelligent on every level.

We also know that DNA emits light, and no one knows why. If someone sits in a room in complete darkness, in front of a camera that is extremely sensitive to light, one can create a photograph of oneself purely from the light of one's DNA. It may be that all of the DNA on this planet is communicating together and that these amazing molecules communicate with signals of light. (It sure seems that way to me under the influence of ayahuasca. More on that later.)

It appears that the essence of what we are is something more like an everlasting field of consciousness than a physical form. We're part of a metaphysical intelligence that has been evolving new life-forms for eons. British biologist Rupert Sheldrake, whom I worked closely with for three years on several research and writing projects, helped to develop the concept of a biological field called a morphogenetic field, which we'll be discussing in more detail later in this book. This concept goes a long way toward helping to explain many mysterious and unexplained reports in science that at first appear paranormal, such as with claims of telepathy, remote viewing, and other forms of psychic phenomena. Maybe even ghosts.

PUTTING THINGS IN PERSPECTIVE

Life has been evolving on Earth for a few billion years, and the earliest fossil records show that human beings first appeared on the scene around a hundred or two hundred million years ago. For the first 60,000 to 160,000 years of our existence, not a whole lot happened. Then, around 40,000 years ago, human culture suddenly appeared. Humanity was on its way to becoming a technological species. No one knows what triggered this explosion of human intelligence, but it happened all at once over the entire planet. All of a sudden humans were painting pictures on cave walls, making crude tools, adorning their bodies with jewelry, and burying their dead with religious objects. Forty thousand years later we have smart phones, the Internet, space shuttles, and endless reruns of *American Idol*.

Most of what we know of human history occurred only in the past four thousand years. "We're as ephemeral as mayflies," Terence McKenna once said. Our time here has been so short. Our senses detect only the smallest slice of the electromagnetic spectrum, which is how we perceive the universe around us, and our brains allow only the tiniest fraction of those signals into our conscious awareness. The models of the world that we create in our minds are extremely limited and highly biased because of our genetics and social/cultural conditioning.

We're pretty much in the dark here. In fact, astrophysicists tell us that the two hundred billion galaxies that are detectable by our best telescopes add up to only about 4 percent of the whole cosmos. Around 96 percent of the universe is composed of dark matter or dark energy that we can't see. Nobody knows what this is, but we know it's there because it massively outweighs all the atoms, in all the stars, in all the galaxies, across the whole detectable range of space. Not to mention the distinct possibility that our universe is merely one out of an infinite number of parallel universes.

From the perspective of cosmic time we've barely had but a moment to try to figure out what's going on here. The past few hundred years of scientific progress have opened up worlds to us, with discoveries our ancestors could hardly have imagined. Science may yet crack the neural code, extend human life indefinitely, and create computers with extraordinary intelligence. Science may help us discover intelligent life elsewhere in the universe, and it may allow us to enhance the powers of our mind. It may ultimately allow us to completely master matter and energy, time and space.

Yet no matter how much our knowledge expands or how godlike our abilities become, there will always be a burning mystery in the center of it all. Even if the ultimate mystery—the origin of our existence—is eternally unsolvable, that doesn't mean that we should stop trying to figure it all out.

Socrates believed that "the aim of life is to know thyself." Searching for the origin of the universe and the genesis of consciousness helps us understand ourselves better—and therein may lie the key to our survival as a species. The process of self-discovery—as individuals and as a species—helps to create a sense of purpose and passion in our lives, and history has shown us, again and again, that life guided by purpose and driven by passion will forever triumph over chaos.

2
Confronting the Mysteries of Science

As a child I loved "Ripley's Believe it or Not!" a syndicated comic-illustrated column about true and bizarre facts from around the world that never failed to baffle and intrigue me. I was always fascinated by strange anomalies, the unusual, fantastic, and weirdly unexplained phenomena that didn't quite fit into conventional thought or scientific theories. It's no coincidence that I currently live in a town whose motto is "Keep Santa Cruz Weird."

When I was young my dad told me that anything is possible, and to this day I suspect that to be true. I'm not sure what I believe to be real exactly, in any ultimate sense, but I'm pretty sure that much of what my brain leads me to believe about reality is an illusion. For example, I realized soon after my first psychedelic experience that the universe isn't really composed of subatomic particles, energy, time, and space, as most physicists would have us believe; rather, it's composed mostly of myths and mystery.

No one really knows how the universe began, what existed before it began, what it's really composed of, how life got started, or what exactly is going on here during our extremely brief flash of existence—although, of course, there's certainly no shortage of people who think they know. No one even understands how our brains are linked with the consciousness that we identify with as ourselves or where we came from. We're about as ignorant as any other species when truly confronted with the vast and unexplainable puzzle of our existence. People who think they know for certain what is going on are surely the most delusional of all.

As my old friend Robert Anton Wilson was fond of saying, "I don't believe anything, but I have my suspicions." This seems like a reasonable and sensible approach to me.

ENCOUNTERING UNEXPLAINED PHENOMENA

I saw a giant dragonfly as a young child. I was out playing by the side of my house in New Jersey when I suddenly spotted a huge dragonfly around three or four feet long, hovering and loudly buzzing about eight feet above my head. It flew ahead of me, circling around the back of the house, and I excitedly chased after it. It was absolutely amazing to see this huge, magical, iridescent creature flying across my backyard, and I desperately tried to catch up with it. Then it turned around the other side of the house, and I watched it suddenly speed off and disappear straight into the sky. Afterward I enthusiastically told everyone about what I had seen, but, of course, no one believed me.

Years later I learned that prehistoric dragonflies really did reach that size. I remember pointing to pictures of them in science books, telling people that that was what I had seen flying in my backyard. Everyone rolled their eyes in disbelief, but to this day I'm convinced of what I saw. Interestingly, Robert Anton Wilson told me that he once saw a giant spider, several feet long, when he was a child.

This was my first encounter with an event that I couldn't easily explain, and it was the beginning of many such occurrences in my life. My life has been filled with an abundance of uncanny synchronicities, unexplained phenomena, and strange events that defy conventional thinking. So rather than just assume I'm crazy, I've long considered our scientific view of the world to be woefully incomplete and inadequate, and I have become relatively comfortable living with a high degree of uncertainty. My many encounters with unusual phenomena have allowed me to become more and more comfortable with the notion that the universe is composed mostly of mystery.

One particularly striking synchroncity happened after I wrote a letter to the national newspaper *USA Today* while tripping on acid. I wrote a letter about President Jimmy Carter's daughter, Amy, who had teamed up with yippie cofounder Abbie Hoffman to protest CIA recruitments on college campuses. I wrote something like, *Rah, rah Amy Carter! That's the American way.* For the next few weeks I checked the paper to see if the editors printed it, but it never showed up. A few months later I received a package of mail from my mom, a bundle of letters that had been sent to my old home address. Among the letters there was a copy of *USA Today,* dated 1987, and I didn't understand why it was there. I almost threw it away. Then I thought, *Hey, maybe my mom sent this to me because my letter was printed in there.* I turned to the letters section of the paper, and, sure enough, there it was.

So I called my mom to thank her for sending this to me, and I said that she should have let me know about my letter being in the paper because I had almost thrown it away. Then she said, "What are you talking about?" I said, "You know, the paper that you just sent me with my letter in it." She had no idea what I was talking about. "Why did you send me that copy of *USA Today*?" I asked her. She replied, "Oh, just because you used to read it when you were living here, and when I was putting together your mail I thought I'd throw it in." She had never sent me a copy of the paper before or since. How does something like this happen? Could it really just be a mere coincidence?

I currently live in the Santa Cruz Mountains of California, where there have been many reported sightings of Bigfoot, or Sasquatch, a supposedly large furry primate that lives in rural areas of North America. Not far down the road from where I live is the Bigfoot Discovery Museum that archives all the sightings, photographs, recordings, and plaster-cast footprints from people who have supposedly encountered the mysterious bipedal creature.

Although as a child I was fascinated by stories of Bigfoot, somewhere during my development the mysterious giant ape got relegated to the part of my brain that deals with Elvis sightings and other extremely unlikely possibilities. I was therefore utterly delighted to meet primate anatomy expert Jeff Meldrum at the Bigfoot Discovery Museum one day, and I spoke with him at length. I learned from him that there really is something to these sightings and it's more than likely that this creature actually exists.

In Meldrum's fascinating book *Sasquatch: Legend Meets Science*—which was praised by primate expert Jane Goodall—Meldrum carefully explores the evidence for this large mysterious primate that supposedly makes its home in the Pacific Northwest. The consistency of the footprints that have been discovered and the minute details that would be extremely difficult to fake, like dermal ridges and bone fractures, are discussed, along with the most compelling evidence of all: the famous Patterson-Gimlin film footage. Contrary to the uninformed claims of vocal skeptics, the large hairy creature in this short film has never been properly identified, and fakery has been ruled out by special-effects experts as well as by experts in primate locomotion. Whatever the creature in this film is, it is most definitely not a human being wearing an ape suit, as there are far too many well-established inconsistencies with this notion.

While I haven't spotted any Sasquatches here in the Santa Cruz Mountains, I keep my eyes open for them every day. I did once hear some mysterious footsteps around my cabin late one night, but I didn't see anything. Nonetheless, I have had some pretty strange events happen here. Here's a bizarre example of an unusual occurrence that I experienced in the Santa Cruz Mountains, one that baffles my conceptual mind and that I'm at loss to explain.

TANTRIC EARTH LIGHTS

One evening in 1999 my girlfriend and I were in my bathroom. The lights were out and it was the early part of the evening, after the sun had gone down. We were kissing and I had my eyes closed. I suddenly noticed that a light was shining directly on my face. I opened my eyes and saw that a bright light beam was coming in through the bathroom window and shining right onto my girlfriend and me. I looked out the window and saw what appeared to be a bright flashlight around twenty or thirty yards away, pointed in the window, directly on us.

At first I thought that it was my landlady out looking for something in the dark, but I became concerned when the focused light beam continued to stay on us. My girlfriend and I stood frozen in front of the window, like a deer caught in a car's headlights, and we looked right into the light beam. Standing there completely naked, I was thinking, *Who in God's name is shining a flashlight in at us?* That's when the really weird phenomena began, for the next twenty to thirty minutes (or what seemed about that length of time).

The bright light beam that had been trained on us began floating around, seemingly weightless, and blinking on and off. There would be total darkness; then several spots on the trees would light up for a few seconds, like small discreet flashes of lightning.

These lightning-like flashes went on for quite some time, and then there were flashes of light in different colors. I saw reds, whites, yellows, and oranges, but my girlfriend told me that she saw other colors as well.

Then we began seeing circles of light with symbols or objects in their center. We saw a circle of yellow light with what appeared to be a bright red lantern in the center. We watched in a state of utter astonishment, fear, and fascination. We just couldn't believe what we were seeing, and it almost seemed as if our emotional reactions were having an effect on the frequency of the lights' blinking. It was so strange, and then it all just suddenly stopped.

When I asked them about it the next day, my neighbors said they didn't see anything unusual. They had no idea what my partner and I saw, and there should have been no one else on the property at that time. I lived in a pretty isolated area, out in the middle of the woods several miles up a steep mountain that is accessible only by car, and mischievous teenagers didn't seem a likely explanation. No people were seen or voices heard.

Then, to top it all off, when we went upstairs into my loft we discovered that far more time had gone by than we could fully account for. The light show that we both witnessed seemed to last less than thirty minutes, yet more than two hours had gone by. After this happened I wasn't able to stop thinking about it for several weeks and asked everyone I knew if they had ever seen anything similar. No one had. Although I had never seen anything like it before in my life, my girl-friend said that she had seen lights like this before in her dreams. Then, after this experience, I had two dreams where I saw similar lights in the trees or a bright light beam shining into my house through the window.

Several weeks after the experience with the lights, while browsing through a used bookstore, I discovered a book by Albert Budden called *Electric UFOs: Fireballs, Electromagnetics and Abnormal States,* which has an interesting section on what are called earth lights. It states that

> during periods of tectonic activity and/or mechanical strain in faults, globes of light were produced which could be of various colors, last for considerable periods of time and had the ability to change shape. Orange and white were the two colors which predom-inated, and one of the mechanisms proposed involved piezoelectric and piezomagnetic process, whereby rock masses, predominantly silicates, produced such energies due to unreleased ground strain. Many different reports of light forms were collected from geologi-cal data around the world, showing that such terrestrial lights could take many different forms, e.g., globes, beams, multicolored points of light, discs, ovoids, etc.

This description of earth lights sounds quite similar to what my partner and I experienced that evening looking out my bathroom window. The Santa Cruz Mountains are riddled with major fault lines, and prior to earthquakes in this area there are often reports of unusual animal behavior. This provides further evidence for what is known as the piezoelectric theory, a leading explanation for earth light reports, which we will be discussing more soon. This theory may also help to explain my girlfriend's and my experience with altered states of consciousness at the time, as electric fields are known to alter neurotransmitter ratios in the brain.

But what caused the light beam to shine directly on us for such a sustained period of time as we were kissing? I couldn't find anything about earth lights that did this. Perhaps the electrically charged, erotic-tantric energies that we were cultivating created a channel or a link of some kind with the electrical energy that manifested as the earth lights. Perhaps our nervous systems were in some type of charged resonance with the electrical field that was being generated by the fault-line pressure on the quartz crystal in the earth's crust. God only knows.

My girlfriend said that she believes the lights that we saw may have been intelligent, alive, and conscious in some way. I have to admit I did have that impression as well, and the tantric earth light theory doesn't discount the possibility that the light was an intelligent entity of some sort. Whatever it was that happened that night we may never know, but it sure was freaking weird.

When I recounted this experience to the late Harvard psychiatric researcher and alien abductee expert John Mack, whom we'll be discussing more later in the book, he was intrigued by it and offered to put me into a relaxed hypnotic state to explore my memory of the event and see if anything else may have happened that I couldn't immediately recall. Unfortunately we never had the opportunity to do this before he died. Although I don't think anything more happened than what I described above, because of John's curiosity I have always wondered. The last time I spoke with John was when I interviewed him for my book *Conversations on the Edge of the Apocalypse.* John died in 2004, when he was accidentally struck by a drunk driver one night in London.

London was where I began my formal study of unexplained phenomena—that which conventional science is at a loss to explain—and where I began to scientifically research what are commonly referred to as psychic abilities.

UNEXPLAINED PHENOMENA IN SCIENCE AND RESEARCH WITH RUPERT SHELDRAKE

My interest in unexplained phenomena led me in 1996 to a close working relationship with the controversial British biologist Rupert Sheldrake, and we worked together on a number of research projects over the next three years involving the unexplained powers of animals. I did the California-based research for two of his bestselling books, *Dogs That Know When Their Owners Are Coming Home* and *The Sense of Being Stared At,* and we coauthored three scientific papers together.

I began working with Rupert because of our common interest in reports of unusual animal behavior prior to earthquakes and also because of our mutual friendship with the late psychedelic historian Nina Graboi, author of *One Foot in the Future.* My interviews with Rupert appear in my books *Mavericks of the Mind* and *Conversations on the Edge of the Apocalypse,* and I had to promise lifelong slavery to my friend Nina for arranging the first interview with Rupert. I did my best to keep my word to Nina, whom I love and miss dearly. I'll be speaking more about her later.

I stayed with Rupert and his family at his home in London for a month when I began working with him on these research projects. We worked closely together, and I got to know him quite well. I learned a lot from Rupert and consider him to be a genius of the highest order. He was one of the most important influences in my life, and he helped to renew the passion I had begun to lose for science when I was in graduate school at USC studying neuroscience. Rupert inspired me enormously in many ways, scientifically and spiritually.

One of Rupert's ideas that particularly intrigues me is the possibility that the laws of physics are not eternally fixed in stone, as many scientists assume. Sheldrake suspects that the laws of physics—like the speed of light or gravitational constants—are merely habits, and they evolve and change over time, just like everything else in the universe.

Rupert has an uncanny ability to draw attention to those annoying anomalies that don't quite fit into our conventional understanding of science and to devise elegantly simple, inexpensive experiments that just about anyone can do, which consistently produce results that conventional science is at a loss to explain. He is also incredibly patient and persistent in pursuing his goals and is unusually charming as a public speaker. I'm convinced that Rupert will go down in history as one of the most important scientists of our times.

Rupert's work strikes a strong nerve in many people. His experiments and popular influence have so infuriated traditional, fundamentalist biologists that they not only denounced his work but have even called out for its burning! John Maddox, the senior editor of *Nature* (one of the most-respected science journals in the world) titled his highly critical review of Sheldrake's first book "A Book for Burning?" (*Nature* also reviewed my book *Mavericks of Medicine* years later, and although they mocked it, at least they didn't recommend burning it.)

The popular evolutionary biologist Richard Dawkins has been one of the most outspoken critics of Sheldrake's work, although he refuses to address critical issues about the actual results and the nature of his assumptions. This is really a shame because many of Dawkins's writings on evolution are otherwise quite brilliant, especially his ideas about memes, or cultural units that replicate themselves like genes and are also subject to the laws of natural selection. When I requested an interview with Dawkins for a previous book and sent him a list of the other people to be included, he replied, "I was going to say yes, but then when I saw that you were interviewing Rupert Sheldrake and Deepak Chopra

I have to decline. How could you?!" Dawkins never replied to any of my messages again.

One of Dawkins's most popular books is about atheism, and it's titled *The God Delusion*. It's an interesting book, as he cleverly points out how ridiculous the myths of most organized religions are, but he fails to even consider the reality of mystical or religious experiences. Sheldrake responded with a book of his own called *The Science Delusion*.

THE UNEXPLAINED POWERS OF ANIMALS

I began researching the unexplained powers of animals as part of my collaboration with Rupert. The research I did with him on the strange behavior that animals sometimes exhibit prior to earthquakes became the backbone for the section on this subject in Rupert's popular book *Dogs That Know When Their Owners Are Coming Home* (which was the bestselling science book in the world for several weeks in fall 2000). I also conducted a number of the experiments for other sections of the book and was responsible for all of the California-based research. This information was updated, with a summary of the earthquake data that has accumulated since *Dogs That Know When Their Owners are Coming Home* was published, in Rupert's more recent book *The Sense of Being Stared At*.

Since I compiled more material about unusual animal behavior prior to earthquakes than Rupert could fit into the section in his book on this subject, I posted much of this material on a website that I built with my friend Joseph Wouk: www.animalsandearthquakes.com, now one of the world's primary sources of information on this subject.

As a result of my research in this area I have received many hundreds of reports from people all over the globe. Almost every time there is a major earthquake somewhere on the planet I receive a number of reports, sometimes a dozen or more. The many anecdotes that I have received have been carefully saved in an ever-growing database.

There is much anecdotal evidence to suggest that some animals have the ability to detect sensory stimuli that humans cannot—even with our most sensitive technological instruments. That many animals have access to a perceptual range exceeding those of humans is scientifically well established, but it also appears that many animals have sensory abilities not currently explained by traditional science. For example, homing pigeons have remarkable abilities to navigate to their desired location in ways that are not fully understood.

Perhaps most significantly, Rupert and colleagues (such as I) have demonstrated how some pets appear to anticipate the arrival of their owner. Regardless of the time of day, some animals appear to sense when their human companion is returning, without receiving any known physical signals. The animal (most often a dog) usually expresses this by waiting in the same spot each time—such as by the door or window— shortly before their owner arrives home. This research is documented in *Dogs That Know When Their Owners Are Coming Home.*

I did a series of experiments for the book that demonstrated that even some birds have the ability to anticipate their owners' arrival in a way that confounds conventional science. I recorded and carefully counted the chirps of cockatiels, which increased in frequency when their human companions began their journey home.

Researching the unexplained powers of animals with Rupert turned out to be an extremely fruitful endeavor. In the initial stages of our research Rupert brought to my attention the following fact, which made a great impression on me: animals have been very carefully studied in laboratory settings as well as in the wild; however, the unique bond that forms between human and pet had never been carefully explored scientifically. This glaringly obvious, empty niche in the history of science, which had eluded so many, seemed to hold great promise.

When I first began my research with Rupert, I already knew that some pet owners believed that they have powerful psychic bonds with their pets and that they sometimes describe their connection with the animal as telepathic, but I had no idea how common this perception was, even though I had experienced it myself. When I was a teenager it seemed as though I was capable of having telepathic conversations with my cat, Fritzy, after I got high on cannabis. I would get stoned while she lay on my chest, purring and looking into my eyes, and we would seemingly converse about all kinds of profound and mundane things.

Dr. Dolittle isn't the only person who claims to be able to communicate with animals. In fact, many ordinary people say that they can do this too, and several books have even been written on the subject. All types of psychic abilities have been attributed to pets by their owners. In addition to telepathy and clairvoyance, some people claim that their pets have precognitive abilities, and, of course, others have noticed that some animals act in peculiar ways just before an earthquake strikes.

In 1990 I witnessed some animals acting strangely just prior to an earthquake in Los Angeles. I was in graduate school at the time, working in the learning and memory lab on the fifth floor of the University of Southern California's Hedco Neurosciences Building. I was working with three other graduate students and three calm rabbits. Suddenly the rabbits became noticeably agitated. They started wildly hopping around in their cages for about five minutes. Then a 5.2 earthquake sent the whole building rolling and swaying.

After my experience with the anxious rabbits I have learned that since the beginning of recorded history virtually every culture in the world has reported observations of unusual animal behavior prior to earthquakes (and, to a lesser extent, volcanic eruptions), but conventional science has never been able to adequately explain the phenomenon. Nonetheless, the Chinese have employed such sightings with some success for hundreds of years as an important part of a nationally orchestrated earthquake warning system.

Perhaps most significantly, on February 4, 1975, the Chinese successfully evacuated the city of Haicheng, based primarily on observations of unusual animal behavior several hours before a 7.3 magnitude earthquake. Ninety percent of the city's structures were destroyed in the quake, but the entire city had been evacuated before it struck. Nearly ninety thousand lives were saved. Since then China has been hit by a number of major quakes for which they were not as prepared, and they have also had some false alarms, so their system is certainly not foolproof. Nevertheless, they have made a remarkable achievement by demonstrating that earthquakes do not always strike without warning.

RESEARCH INTO UNUSUAL ANIMAL BEHAVIOR
PRIOR TO EARTHQUAKES

Helmut Tributsch's classic work on the subject of earthquakes and unusual animal behavior, *When the Snakes Awake,* details numerous consistent accounts of the phenomenon from all over the world. Although these behavior patterns are well documented, most geologists whom I have spoken with at the United States Geological Survey (USGS) don't take them very seriously. The official word from the USGS and the National Earthquake Prediction Evaluation Council is that no form of earthquake prediction—observations of unusual animal behavior included—performs better than chance.

This is ironic and unfortunate, because the USGS itself funded a Stanford Research Institute (SRI) study for several years back in the early 1980s that showed promising results. Inspired by China's success, in 1975 William Kautz (whom I interviewed for my animal and earthquake website) and Leon Otis created Project Earthquake Watch. For the project they recruited hundreds of volunteers from all over California to observe their animals for any unusual behavior and to call a toll-free hotline to record their observations. Kautz and Otis got significant results—that is, before some earthquakes more people reported unusual animal behavior—but the USGS stopped funding the study for reasons no one whom I've spoken to seems to know or really care about.

The notion that odd animal behavior can help people predict earthquakes is perceived by most traditional geologists in the West as folklore or an old wives' tale and is often cast into the same boat as sightings of poltergeists, Elvis, and the Loch Ness Monster. The ancient Greeks, on the other hand, considered an understanding of the relationship between unusual animal behavior and earthquakes to be an esoteric form of secret knowledge.

In ancient Persia (now Iran) wise men predicted earthquakes using a forecasting process that included digging wells, looking at the moon and stars, and observing animal behavior. That such strong support for the application of this knowledge still exists in the East—in long-lived civilizations like those in China and Japan—is testimony to the reality of the phenomenon, as they have witnessed many more earthquakes in their long histories than has a comparatively young country like the United States.

But not all Western geologists are closed-minded with regard to the phenomenon. James Berkland, a retired USGS geologist from Santa Clara County, California, claims to be able to predict earthquakes with greater than a 75 percent accuracy rate, simply by counting the number of lost-pet ads in the daily newspaper classifieds and correlating this relationship to the lunar and tide cycles. This maverick geologist has been meticulously saving and counting lost-pet ads for many years. Berkland says that the number of missing dogs and cats goes up significantly for as long as two weeks prior to an earthquake. I interviewed Berkland and spent many hours in the local library rolling through microfilm collections of *The San Jose Mercury News* counting lost-pet ads in an (inconclusive) attempt to check out Berkland's claims.

Gravitational variations due to lunar cycles, he says, create "seismic windows" of greater earthquake probability. When the number of missing pets also suddenly rises, then—bingo—a quake is likely to happen. Berkland said that he thinks the USGS won't accept unusual animal data because it doesn't jibe with their current scientific paradigm and hypotheses. (Researchers who attempt earthquake prediction are often lumped by traditional geologists into the same category as fortune-tellers and scam artists.) It is not surprising, then, to hear that Berkland was suspended from his position as Santa Clara County geologist for claiming to predict earthquakes—such as the 1989 Loma Prieta quake in northern California, which was preceded by numerous reports of odd animal behavior.

Unusual behavior is difficult to define, and determining if there is a characteristic behavior is not a simple, clear-cut process, although some distinct patterns have emerged. For example, an intense fear that appears to make some animals cry and bark for hours and others flee in panic has been reported often. Equally characteristic is the apparent opposite effect of wild animals appearing confused and disoriented and losing their usual fear of people. Some other common observations are that animals appear agitated, excited, nervous, or overly aggressive, or seem to be trying to burrow or hide.

In 1996 I conducted a telephone survey of Santa Cruz County households to find out how many people have observed unusual animal behavior prior to earthquakes. Out of the two hundred people randomly selected from the phone book, 15 percent told me they had observed an animal acting oddly before an earthquake. When I conducted a telephone survey of Los Angeles County the following year I found precisely the same figure: 15 percent out of two hundred. Some common observations were animals appearing frightened, agitated, panic-stricken, excited, or confused.

A number of people found that their ordinarily mellow cats suddenly darted off and hid or paced around crying for a few minutes before the quake. I was told of goats and horses leaping around wildly, noisy birds suddenly becoming silent, or a whole flock of seagulls taking off all at once just before an earthquake. A few people told me that they noticed the number of roadkill increasing for several days before a quake. A lot of people mentioned dogs vanishing or barking uncontrollably.

One Santa Cruz woman told me her neighbor's dog jumped a fence just before the 1989 Loma Prieta quake in northern California, then the dog sat on her daughter through the quake, as though trying to protect her. Other stories are just plain bizarre. One woman said that her cat did a backflip off her balcony. Another woman reported that her cat leaped out of a two-story window shortly before a quake.

Although the majority of accounts pertain to dogs and cats, there are also many stories about other types of animals in the wild, on farms, and in zoos, including horses, cows, deer, goats, opossums, rats, chickens, and other birds. I haven't heard any reports of Sasquatches acting strangely prior to earthquakes, but unusual behavior has been reported in many other species, including fish, jellyfish, reptiles, and even insects. Deep-sea fish, for example, have been caught close to the surface of the ocean on numerous occasions around Japan prior to earthquakes. Before the giant waves of a tsunami slammed into the Sri Lanka and India coastlines in 2005, elephants seemed to know what was about to happen and fled to the safety of higher ground.

Some fish—catfish in particular—are reputed to become especially agitated before earthquakes and at times have been reported to actually leap out of the water onto dry land. Snakes have been known to leave their underground places of hibernation in the middle of the winter prior to quakes only to be found frozen on the surface of the snow. Mice are commonly reported to appear dazed before quakes and allow themselves to be easily captured by hand. Homing pigeons are said to take much longer to navigate to their destination prior to earthquakes.

Bees have been seen evacuating their hive in a panic minutes before an earthquake and then not returning until fifteen minutes after the quake ends. Even creatures such as millipedes, leeches, squids, and ants have been reported to exhibit abnormal behavior prior to earthquakes.

These strange behaviors generally occur anywhere from moments to weeks in advance of a quake. Most of the people I have spoken with who have witnessed this phenomenon observed strange behavior within twenty-four hours of a quake, although some observations occurred more than a week before the quake struck. Berkland has suggested that there are possibly two primary precursory earthquake signals: one several weeks before, and the other one just moments before the quake. Many reports appear to confirm this.

A number of theories have been proposed to explain why animals sometimes act in peculiar ways prior to earthquakes and what the precursory signals that the animals are picking up on might be. The scientific theories that have been proposed to explain this phenomenon generally fall into six major categories: ultrasound vibrations, magnetic field fluctuations, electrical-field variations, piezoelectric airborne ions, brain changes, and precognition, which I discuss in detail on my website www.animalsandearthquakes.com. However, the theory that makes the most sense to me is electrical-field theory.

ELECTRICAL-FIELD THEORY

Fish are known to have a high degree of sensitivity to variations in electric fields, and this appears to be an important clue for understanding how animals react to pre-earthquake signals. The surface of the Earth has a constant electrical field, and because telluric current variations (natural electric currents flowing near the Earth's surface) have also been noted before some earthquakes, it has been suggested that this may be what the fish are reacting to. To test this hypothesis Motoji Ikeya and his colleagues at Osaka University in Japan have done numerous studies where they exposed a variety of animals—including minnows, catfish, eels, and earthworms—to a weak electrical field.

Ikeya's laboratory experiments were conducted to see if exposure to a weak electrical field could elicit the pre-earthquake animal behaviors— what the Japanese call Seismic Animal Anomalous Behavior (SAAB). Ikeya's experiments produced interesting results. When the current was applied fish showed panic reactions, and earthworms moved out of the soil and swarmed. An interview that I did with Ikeya appears on my website.

Unlike their American counterparts, some Japanese researchers take SAAB research quite seriously. A group of Japanese researchers have even gone so far as to do genetic experiments to see if they can find specific genes that encode for a sensitivity to pre-earthquake signals, which would make some animal breeds more sensitive than others. (However, these studies by individual Japanese scientists do not necessarily reflect the general attitude of most contemporary seismologists in Japan. When I interviewed Professor Junzo Kasahara, a prominent geophysicist at the Earthquake Prediction Research Institute at the University of Tokyo, he told me that most seismologists in Japan don't take the SAAB research that seriously.)

Helmut Tributsch has suggested that a piezoelectric effect may be responsible for triggering the pre-earthquake behaviors in animals, and this explanation seems significantly more plausible than the other explanations I've heard. This theory makes sense because of the following facts. When certain crystals, such as quartz, are arranged in a way that pressure is applied along particular portions of the crystal's axes, the distribution of positive and negative ions can shift slightly.

In this way pressure changes to produce electrical charging of the crystal's surfaces. On average the Earth's crust consists of 15 percent quartz, and in certain areas it can be as high as 55 percent.

According to Tributsch the piezoelectric effect of the quartz is capable of generating enough electrical energy to account for the creation of airborne ions before and during an earthquake. This electrostatic charging of aerosol particles may be what the animals are reacting to, and this phenomenon may also help to explain the mechanics behind the earthlight show that my girlfriend and I witnessed. Because some animals have also been observed acting frightened prior to thunderstorms and are known to flee areas or show signs of distress before a storm arrives, it may be that they have evolved a sensitivity to electrical changes in their environment.

THE NERVOUS SYSTEM AND ELECTRIC FIELDS

Some people say that they feel an uncomfortable pressure in their head or a persistent headache that lasts for weeks and then suddenly vanishes moments before an earthquake strikes. Because magnetite has been found in some animal brains, Berkland thinks it is possible that animals may be reacting to their own headaches caused by changes in the Earth's electromagnetic field. He said that a dog was observed chewing on willow bark—the plant from which aspirin is derived—prior to an earthquake, and he believes that this was an attempt by the dog to self-medicate the headache.

Berkland also told me that some people with multiple sclerosis, a disease caused by improper insulation around the electrically conductive fibers of the nervous system, experience an increase in symptoms weeks before an earthquake. Because the nervous system is an electrochemical system it doesn't seem surprising that geologically based electrical-field changes would disrupt its functioning.

Besides unusual animal behavior, other mysterious phenomena are often connected with earthquakes. The regular eruptions of geysers have been interrupted. Well levels have been reported to change, or the water in them has been known to become cloudy. Magnets have been said to temporarily lose their power. Many people report that there is suddenly an unexplainable stillness in the air and that everything around them becomes completely silent. Unusual fog has been reported, and strange lights are often seen glowing from the earth, as I described earlier in my section on earth lights.

These phenomena are all consistent with the notion that odd animal behavior may result from changes in the Earth's electromagnetic field or the release of electrically charged particles from intense pressure on crystalline rock. It's interesting that a number of people claim to have sighted UFOs hovering around earthquake sites. Even more puzzling to explain are the reports of unusual animal behavior prior to so-called alien abduction experiences, which Karen Wesolowski, executive director of the Program for Extraordinary Experience Research (PEER), told me about. (PEER is an organization that was founded by the late John Mack to study and support people who believe they have been abducted by alien beings.)

The UFO sightings are probably caused by something similar to the earth lights I described earlier, a phenomenon called selsmoatmospheric luminescence, in which the release of electrically charged particles from the Earth causes auras and lights to be seen. This and other electrical anomalies, like interference in radio and television broadcasts, seem best explained by the electrical changes that occur prior to earthquakes.

DISRUPTIONS IN THE MIND FIELD

A possible explanation for the psychological effects underlying the strange animal behavior arises from the fact that electrically charged ionic particles have been shown to change neurotransmitter (chemical messenger) ratios in animal brains. More specifically, electrically charged ionic particles have been shown to alter serotonin (a neurotransmitter responsible for neural inhibition) levels in animal brains. Because charged ions may be released prior to some earthquakes, it has been suggested that this may explain the two seemingly contradictory behavior patterns discussed earlier, where normally calm pets seem to become frightened and wild animals often appear to lose their sense of fear.

Serotonin levels in the brain help to mediate an animal's fear response. This is why serotonin reuptake–inhibiting antidepressants like Prozac are prescribed for people with social anxiety. By increasing serotonin availability in the brain, the emotion of fear is reduced. Pre-earthquake electrical-field changes may affect neurotransmitter levels in different species of animals' brains in different ways, and this may account for the difference in reactions between wild and domesticated animals. However, it does appear that serotonin is, at least, one of the primary neurochemical variables that is altered prior to earthquakes. There could be others.

These neurotransmitter changes could possibly help to explain another related phenomenon. I've noticed that earthquakes, like solar eclipses, sometimes trigger an intense consciousness-altering experience in people. People often feel energized, emotionally open, and acutely sensitive following earthquakes. Powerful bonding experiences often occur between people in the aftermath of a quake. It's interesting that people almost seem like they're under the influence of MDMA (Ecstasy, which floods the brain with serotonin) after earthquakes. Earthquake victims frequently walk around after the quake in a euphoric daze, hugging one another and expressing feelings of love.

Although this is likely to be true for any natural disaster that people share, there may be more going on. Subjectively, earthquake experiences often take on dreamlike qualities or have a sense of unreality about them. Perhaps this is because our most cherished notion of what is safe and solid in the world—the very ground upon which we rest—becomes wobbly and unstable. Our whole sense of reality is shaken with the earth, as one is suddenly lifted out of the mundane and thrust into the center of what seems to be an immensely important drama. This experience can be quite intense, so it's not inconceivable to suppose that geologically generated electrical signals stimulate our nervous systems in ways that heighten this experience by altering our neurotransmitter levels.

It appears that electrical-field effects like these are merely part of a spectrum of field effects that biology has yet to recognize.

MORPHIC-FIELD THEORY AND THE PRESENCE OF THE PAST

Rupert Sheldrake's theory for explaining the unexplained powers of animals, and many other mysterious phenomena in science, is based on his hypothesis of formative causation, which helps to unravel one of the biggest mysteries in biology: the process of morphogenesis, or how new life-forms develop and come into being.

Central to Sheldrake's theory of morphogenesis is the idea that there are no fixed laws of nature, only habits that change and evolve over time, just like everything else in the universe. The speed of light, for example, may not be fixed in stone as physicists believe, and it could vary as the universe evolves. Measurements of the speed of light over time actually support this notion, but scientists have always assumed that the instruments were mistaken and that the laws of nature are fixed and unchangeable. But there is no good reason to assume that the laws of nature are immutable when everything else in the universe is dynamically changing and evolving.

Currently conventional biologists assume that the entire three-dimensional organization process known as morphogenesis is somehow encoded in our DNA. According to Rupert, this seems impossible as a biological organism is simply too complex for this, and he thinks that a morphic field is necessary to guide the process.

According to Rupert a morphic field is "a field within and around a 'morphic unit' which organizes its characteristic structure and pattern of activity." A *field* in physics is defined as "a nonmaterial region of influence," and a *morphic unit* could be anything that changes form over time—a quartz crystal, a potato plant, a human being, a group of human beings, a biosphere, a galaxy, or even a universe. A morphic field underlies the form and behavior of morphic units at all levels of complexity, Rupert says, and this term includes biological, behavioral, social, cultural, and mental fields.

Rupert thinks that these fields are shaped and stabilized by a process known as morphic resonance, from previous similar morphic units that were under the influence of fields of the same kind. In other words, every flower is resonating like a tuning fork with all of its previous botanical relatives. As a result these fields consequently contain a kind of cumulative memory and tend to become increasingly habitual, so the more something happened in the past, the more likely it is to happen in the future.

Morphic resonance is the influence of previous structures on the activity of subsequent similar structures by activity-organized morphic fields. A morphogenetic field is a type of morphic field—a biological field in particular—that is defined as "a nonmaterial region of influence that guides the structural development of organic forms." These fields, Rupert says, are akin to the established fields known to exist in physics.

I asked Terence McKenna what he thought about applying morphic theory to the use of new psychedelic drugs that don't have a long history of shamanic usage and if he thought that new morphic fields of consciousness could be created this way. He replied:

> Possibly, although I don't know how you grab the morphic field of a new designer drug. For instance, I'll speak to my own experience, which is ketamine. My impression of ketamine was it's like a brand-new skyscraper, all the walls, all the floors are carpeted in white, all the drinking fountains work, the elevators run smoothly, the fluorescent lights recede endlessly in all directions down the hallways. It's just that there's nobody there. There's no office machinery, there's no hurrying secretaries, there's no telephones, it's just this immense, empty structure waiting. Well, I can't move into a sixty-story office building, I have only enough stuff to fill a few small rooms, so it gives me a slightly spooked-out feeling to enter into these empty morphic fields. If you take mushrooms, you know, you're climbing on board a starship manned by every shaman who ever did it in front of you, and this is quite a crew, and they've really pulled some stunts over the millennia, and it's all there, the tapes to be played, but the designer things should be very cautiously dealt with.

We'll be discussing ketamine more later, but Rupert has devised a number of simple experiments that have been replicated many hundreds of times, which appear to confirm his radical theory of morphogenesis and his explanation for psychic phenomena. To test some of these experiments yourself, see Rupert's book *Seven Experiments That Could Change the World,* or visit his website: www.sheldrake.org.

ESP AND PSYCHIC PHENOMENA

Through Rupert, I met his colleague Dean Radin, who has been researching psychic phenomena at prestigious universities and major research centers since the beginning of his career as a psychologist, with consistent, repeatable, and extremely compelling results. He is now considered one of the world's experts on the subject.

Few people are aware that there have been numerous, carefully controlled scientific experiments with telepathy, psychokinesis, remote viewing, and other types of psychic phenomena, which have consistently produced compelling, statistically significant results that conventional science is at a loss to explain. It's also interesting to note that many people have reported experiencing meaningful telepathic communications and remote-viewing abilities with ayahuasca and other psychedelics, not to mention a wide range of paranormal events and synchronicities that seem extremely difficult to explain by means of conventional reasoning.

A questionnaire study conducted by psychologist Charles Tart of 150 experienced marijuana users found that 76 percent believed in extrasensory perception (ESP), with frequent reports of experiences while intoxicated that were interpreted as psychic. Psychiatrist Stanislav Grof, M.D., and psychologist Stanley Krippner have collected numerous anecdotes about psychic phenomena that were reported by people under the influence of psychedelics, and several small scientific studies have explored how LSD, psilocybin, and mescaline might affect telepathy and remote viewing.

For example, according to psychologist Jean Millay, in 1997 students at the University of Amsterdam in the Netherlands did a study to establish whether the use of psilocybin could influence remote viewing. This was a small experiment, with only twelve test subjects, but the results of this research indicated that those subjects who were under the influence of psilocybin achieved a success rate of 58.3 percent, which was statistically significant.

In Dean Radin's books *The Conscious Universe* and *The Entangled Mind* he summarizes the past century's research into psychic phenomena, which has largely been hidden from the public, and I did a fascinating in-depth interview with him for my book *Conversations on the Edge of the Apocalypse.*

Dean is currently the senior scientist at the Institute of Noetic Sciences, a unique research institute cofounded by NASA astronaut Edgar Mitchell, which is designed to conduct research on human potentials and institute programs that include "extended human capacities," "integral health and healing," and "emerging worldviews." The Institute of Noetic Sciences helped to fund a portion of the research that Rupert and I did together. To find out more about this extraordinary organization see www.noetic.org.

When I interviewed physicist Nick Herbert for my book *Mavericks of the Mind,* I asked him if he thought that the nonlocal, instantaneous information transfer that is known to occur with subatomic particles due to Bell's theorem might help to explain telepathy. Because everything that has ever been in contact is forevermore connected, and because everything in the universe was initially bound together before the Big Bang, it seems that Bell's theorem might offer a plausible explanation for how two minds can communicate without any known sensory signals. Herbert replied, "Yes, quantum entanglement can help to explain telepathy. But what explains the lack of telepathy?"

Once one understands the basics of quantum theory it seems that the lack of telepathy in the world is perhaps a bigger mystery than mind-to-mind communication. Understanding psychic phenomena may require us to view the nature of reality, space, and time in a whole new way.

ALTERED PERCEPTIONS OF TIME

It may be that different animal species perceive time in different ways. What we perceive as the current moment, right now, is actually a slice of time in the space-time continuum that is composed of a certain thickness—how far it extends into the past and future, as right now is experienced. For most people, most of the time, this is about a second or less. However, it may be that other animal species have a different or more expanded sense of the present moment than we do, a larger slice of the space-time continuum, that possibly extends further into the past and future than ours normally does, and this may help to explain why some dogs are reputed to be able to anticipate their owner's arrival.

One of the most commonly reported experiences with cannabis and psychedelics is a sense of time dilation; time tends to go by unusually slowly when people are high or tripping. People are often astonished to discover that only a few minutes have passed after a subjective experience on psychedelics that felt like hours, or, in the case with DMT, even a whole lifetime can seem to be condensed into just a few minutes of normal human clock-measured time.

I've heard fascinating reports of people doing the dissociative anesthetic DXM and then actually transforming into another person, living in another reality, for weeks—going to sleep, waking up, and going to work for many days—only to suddenly snap back into this reality and discover that only a few hours of Earth time had passed. As Einstein demonstrated mathematically, time is indeed relative, depending on the perspective of the observer.

Additionally many people report that they can actually feel the psychological effects of a psychedelic drug or plant hours before they take it, as though waves from the future psychedelic experience were traveling backward in time to the present moment. This phenomenon can be used as a way to preview the experience before taking the drug so that people can more easily decide if they are properly prepared to trip that day or not.

Radin did a series of fascinating experiments known as presentiment research, which provide us with fascinating insight into the mysterious phenomenon of how we perceive time. Radin had his subjects hooked up to a galvanic skin-response measuring device, which records changes in the electrical conductivity of one's skin over time, and this has been correlated with strong emotional reactions. In fact, this is the basis for using polygraph tests as lie-detection devices.

Radin's subjects were comfortably seated in front of a computer screen, which randomly displayed a series of photographic images. The majority of images were pleasant, neutral images of natural scenery or smiling people, but some of the images were inserted specifically because of their significant shock value. Erotically charged sexual images and disturbing violent images were interspersed with the neutral and pleasant scenes.

Predictably, when the subjects saw a shocking image there was a significant shift in their electrical skin conductivity. However, the results clearly showed that the spikes in people's electrical skin-conductivity patterns began to change several seconds before they actually viewed the shocking image on the computer monitor. Somehow their bodies already knew what to expect before they actually saw the image on the screen. These results have been independently replicated at numerous labs around the world, and Nobel Prize winner Kary Mullis participated as a subject in Radin's experiments and was genuinely perplexed by the results.

The late ethnobotanist Terence McKenna had some truly fascinating and original ideas about the nature of time that have influenced my thinking a great deal, and his controversial timewave theory may shed some light on our understanding of time. McKenna envisioned time as a wave, with a beginning point and an end point, and he developed the notion that the acceleration of novelty in human history is leading us to a mathematically determined point of "infinite novelty" where our imaginations will eventually become externalized as our minds turn themselves inside out and everything becomes possible.

The end of time, McKenna proposes, is the end of a cumulative process of ever-increasing novelty where it eventually reaches a point of infinite frequency and density. When I interviewed Terence about this he playfully told me that he thought that the ultimate goal of human evolution was "a good party." However, his timewave theory provides a more comprehensive summary of his views on where time is leading human evolution, and we'll be discussing this in greater detail in the next chapter.

I asked physicist Nick Herbert what he thought about the possibility of time travel and if he thought it was actually possible to build a time machine. He replied with step-by-step instructions.

I think that there are about half a dozen options for faster-than-light travel, but the two I would bet on are the space-warp, and the quantum connection. The former is based upon the ability to warp Einsteinian space-time. You can make short cuts in space-time, and essentially travel faster than light. We don't know how to do this yet, but the equations of general relativity allow it. So it's not forbidden by physics. We may have to use black holes or something like tongs made out of black holes. It would take that kind of thing. Interestingly, when my book *Faster Than Light* came out in November of 1988, the same week it came out, there was a paper by three guys from CalTech in the journal *Physical Review Letters*. The article was about a way to make a time machine, using warped space-time. It was actual instructions on how to do it. We can't do it yet—but here's, in principle, how to do it. There are these quantum worm holes coming out of the quantum vacuum. They're little connections between distant places in space-time. They're not so distant actually, as the distances involved are smaller than atomic dimensions. So you have to find out how to expand these worm holes, to make them connect larger more distant parts of space and time. But that's a detail. These worm holes are continually coming out of the quantum vacuum, popping back in again, and they're unstable. Even if you could go into one of these, it would close up before you could transverse it, unless you could go faster than light. So, the argument was about how to stabilize quantum worm holes. The way you do that is you have to have some energy that's less than nothing, some negative energy, which is less than the vacuum. In classical physics that would be impossible—energy that's less than nothing. Every time you do something you always have positive energy. But there's something called the Casimer force in quantum physics, which is an example of negative energy. So you thread these worm holes with this negative energy, and it props them open. So then you can use these things as time tunnels. This article was prompted by Carl Sagan's book *Contact*. Sagan got in touch with these physicists, who were experts on gravity, and asked if there was anything that he needed to know, because in his book *Contact* there were tunnels that go to the star Vega, I believe. You sit in this chair, you go through this time tunnel, and a few seconds later you're in Vega. That's definitely faster than light, as Vega is some tens of light-years away. So these aliens have mastered this time tunnel technology. Carl Sagan asked these guys if this was possible, and they said "Well, we'll think about it." So they came up with this actual scientific paper on how one might really build a time tunnel, like Carl Sagan's. So here's a situation where science fiction inspired science.

In his book *Critical Path,* Buckminster Fuller points out that the time it takes for human knowledge to double has been logarithmically decreasing since the beginning of recorded history. Time becomes compressed as the accumulation of information speeds up, and more and more happens in less and less time. According to technology expert Ray Kurzweil, this acceleration of accumulated knowledge is leading us into a technological "singularity" where computer intelligence surpasses human intelligence, nanotechnology will make almost anything possible, and future predictions beyond that point become meaningless.

It is generally thought that at the beginning of the Big Bang, and inside some black holes (or collapsed stars), gravitational fields become infinite, and this causes the known laws of physics—both general relativity and quantum mechanics—to break down. In astrophysics this is known as a *singularity.*

Many physicists suspect that singularities are portals into whole new universes where new laws of physics may operate. This seems like a good poetic metaphor for what the human species appears to be heading into—a point where all the previous rules no longer apply, or don't apply in the same ways.

This idea dovetails with McKenna's visionary notion that the acceleration of novelty in human history is leading us to an unprecedented stage in our evolutionary development where our inner minds and consensual reality indistinguishably blur together, and a new worldview and unified state emerges that transcends the obvious limits of either component in the duality. That is, if we don't destroy ourselves first.

3
The Future Evolution of the Human Species

We can aspire to reach any kind of higher state of evolution only if we survive as a species. So another one of the questions that I've asked many of the people I interviewed was about whether they thought our species will survive much longer, and, if so, how we might evolve in the future. I think this is one of the most important questions we can ask ourselves.

WILL THE HUMAN SPECIES SURVIVE?

We are living in a time that is marked by one of the most widespread mass extinctions in the history of our planet. Conservation biologists tell us that climate change, habitat destruction, ozone depletion, toxic chemicals, and invasive or infectious species are driving back biodiversity on this planet 65 million years, to the lowest level of vitality since the end of the age of the dinosaurs. During that period at least half of all species went extinct, more or less overnight.

When I interviewed physicist and author Peter Russell, he told me: "The same thing is happening right now; species are becoming extinct at a fantastic rate. It's suggested that three species an hour are becoming extinct in the world."

If present trends continue half of all species on Earth will be extinct in less than a hundred years. While it's natural for species to go extinct, and, in fact, the majority of species that have lived on this planet have gone extinct (only about one in a thousand species that ever lived on Earth is still living today), there have only been five other periods in our planet's 4.5-billion-year history where there have been extinctions on the scale that we are currently witnessing.

Mass extinctions, defined as "episodes when an exceptional global decline in biodiversity takes place," affect a broad range of life-forms over a relatively short period of time. Various explanations have been given for these five previous mass extinctions in our planet's history, such as the effects of glaciation, ultraviolet radiation from the sun after gamma rays from a supernova explosion destroyed the Earth's ozone layer, or the widespread climatic impact of an asteroid striking the Earth.

When I interviewed Nobel Prize–winning chemist Kary Mullis he told me he believes the ever-present possibility of an asteroid colliding with the Earth poses the biggest threat to the human species. Our solar system is filled with massive asteroids, and their ever-shifting paths collide with orbiting planets on occasion. One such collision may have ended the reign of the dinosaurs 65 million years ago. According to Mullis it could happen again at any time.

However, the driving force behind the present episode of mass extinctions is not due to a wayward asteroid but, rather, to the impact of a single species—*Homo sapiens.* Human actions have resulted in the widespread loss, fragmentation, and poisoning of natural habitats and the gross disruption of the numerous intricate natural processes that affect the delicate balance of our planet's ecosystems. Humanity could very well be driving itself into extinction.

A 2004 U.S. Pentagon study titled "An Abrupt Climate Change Scenario and Its Implications for United States National Security" warns of the possibility of global warming pushing the planet into a new ice age. According to the Pentagon report the question is not if abrupt climate change will happen, but when. The study goes on to describe a world where riots and wars over food and drinkable water become common place, as 400 million people are forced to migrate from uninhabitable areas.

THE MIGHTY NEW SUPERTECHNOLOGIES

If these present environmental trends aren't alarming enough, there are new technologies emerging on the horizon. Many of the new technologies that we are developing are double-edged swords. Bill Joy, chief scientist for Sun Microsystems, proposed in his widely reprinted *Wired* magazine article "Why the Future Doesn't Need Us" that biotechnology, nanotechnology, and robotics may result in the creation of unnatural entities that can self-replicate beyond human control. While nanotechnology and robotics may allow us to create marvels of medical science that will extend human life indefinitely and tap in to a vast abundance of new resources, there are much darker possibilities as well.

When contemplating the power of these mighty new supertechnologies one can't help but think of the warnings from science-fiction movies. One immediately thinks of HAL, the psychotic computer in *2001: A Space Odyssey* and the deadly super-robots in *The Matrix* and *Terminator* films. And who can forget the haunting slogan from *Westworld,* Michael Crichton's 1973 movie about robots gone berserk? "Nothing can possibly go wrong . . . go wrong . . . go wrong."

The late neuroscientist and consciousness explorer John C. Lilly once warned that superintelligent machines from the future—the Solid State Entities—represented the largest threat to organic life on the planet. (However, when I asked John about this a few years later he said that his concern about the Solid State Entities was just his way of getting in touch with his teeth and bones.)

Even more unthinkable than machines evolving beyond human control or a nanotechnological accident is the possibility of misguided individuals deliberately using these powerful technologies to further their nefarious agendas. A nation-state government blinded by rage or an angry terrorist group could do far more destruction with nanotechnology than with a nuclear bomb or a deadly weaponized virus. Like the protoplasmic creature that arrived on a meteorite from outer space in the movie *The Blob,* self-replicating nanomachines could reduce all organic life on this planet to a giant mass of "gray goo," as nanotechnology expert Eric Drexler warns in his book *Engines of Creation.*

Ecological disasters, technological malfunctions, and terrorist nightmares aside, there are some people who simply believe that an end to humanity's reign on Earth is inevitable. They say that humanity lies on the brink of Armageddon, the end of the world is near, and that we are currently witnessing the Last Days prophesied in the Judeo-Christian Bible. However, in Yuri Rubinsky and Ian Wiseman's eye-opening book, *A History of the End of the World,* they clearly demonstrate how some people have proclaimed that the end was near throughout all of human history.

Nonetheless, only in the past few decades have we developed the technology to actually drive ourselves into extinction, and the current situation in the world has truly never seemed more dire. On this planet there are thousands of thermonuclear bombs and vast stores of genetically modified pathogens that have the capacity to end life as we know it. Every day the U.S. military is working to produce faster, lighter, deadlier weapons. Meanwhile the political situation appears to be growing more chaotic and unpredictable every day.

Some of the people I have interviewed over the years have spoken with great urgency and concern about the dangers. For example, when I spoke with U.S. foreign-policy critic Noam Chomsky he warned:

> We've come very close to terminal nuclear war a number of times. It's kind of a miracle that the species has escaped in fact. And those threats are increasing. For example, the development and the expansion of military systems into space—with highly destructive space-based offensive weapons, that are probably on hair-trigger alert—is almost a guarantee of devastation, if only by accident.

EVE OF THE APOCALYPSE OR DAWN OF A RENAISSANCE?

Despite all of the difficult challenges that we face in the world today, most of the people I have interviewed over the years told me that they don't believe the human species is headed toward extinction, and I share this view. I have too much faith in human ingenuity and our evolving intelligence.

As science-fiction author Bruce Sterling told me:

It would be difficult to exterminate a broadly spread species. It's like asking, Do you think that every rat will be gone in the next hundred years? I mean, we're at least as inventive as they are.

Celebrated stage magician Jeff McBride echoed this by saying:

I think we're just a bit smarter than cockroaches, and look how long they've lasted.

But rats and cockroaches don't make nuclear weapons. Although everyone whom I spoke with recognized the dangers, most expressed cautious optimism. For example, technology expert Ray Kurzweil told me:

We have enough nuclear weapons to destroy all mammalian life on the planet . . . yet when nuclear weapons were exploded in the 1940s, who would have predicted that, nearly sixty years later, not a single other atomic weapon would have been used in anger? . . . There's a lot of things that we don't like about human behavior, and yet we have actually been successful in not only not destroying the world, but in not even having a single weapon go off. Now, we can't say, "Okay, we solved that problem," because we still have the enormous danger. But that does give us some cause for optimism.

As I mentioned earlier, some of the people I interviewed actually expressed great optimism about the future—such as Robert Anton Wilson, who told me shortly before he died that he was even more optimistic than he had been thirty years prior.

> . . . Because I don't think politics has as much importance as most people imagine. The real changes occur first in pure science, then in technology, then in social forms; the politicians then run around in front of the parade and pretend they're leading it—like Al Gore claiming he invented the Internet. If you only look at Dubya and Osama, the world looks like a Dark Age madhouse, but look at biotech, computer science, and space colonies, and a much more hopeful scenario dawns.

Despite all the escalating chaos, confusion, and ever-increasing darkness in the world today, I am also now more optimistic than ever before about the future evolution of our species. There are a number of reasons for this upbeat perspective.

First of all, no one has ever been able to successfully predict the future, because there are simply too many factors interacting and too many unknown variables. Yet people have been predicting doom and gloom since the beginning of recorded history—despite the fact that most things have been getting measurably better and better for us. In Matt Ridley's wonderful book *The Rational Optimist,* he clearly shows how we have been progressively improving virtually every aspect of our lives since the beginning of recorded history, almost no matter how one measures this.

According to Ridley, ideas "have sex" with one another, and they produce "children," offspring ideas that follow a process of natural selection. Because of this process our collective intelligence has been growing at an ever-increasing pace, and Ridley believes that it will save us from our current global crisis, just as it always has in the past. Ridley examines human ingenuity, health, longevity, violence, wealth, transportation, communication, the trade of commodities, and the environment from a historical point of view, which allows us to see our current planetary crisis in a new and decidedly more cheerful light.

Just as there have always been people who thought that the end of the world was near, so too, it seems, have there always been people who have proclaimed the opposite—that humanity is on the brink of a New Age, a planetary awakening, or a quantum leap in evolution. The Human Potential Movement and a lot of pop mystics claim that we are evolving into a higher species and headed into a golden age of enlightenment. There is nothing new about these predictions— the mystical artist and poet William Blake and the cofounder of the Theosophical Society Madame Helena Blavatsky began talking about the dawning of a New Age in the 1800s. The Italian philosopher Giordano Bruno made similar claims in the 1500s, as have many others throughout history.

Ironically, it is the very same technologies—nanotechnology, artificial intelligence, and advanced robotics—that give us the power to reduce all organic life on the planet to a puddle of gray goo, which also hold the keys to a utopian world free of aging, disease, poverty, and possibly even death. With incredible speed, replicating molecular nanomachines capable of precisely sequencing atoms could be programmed to repair any type of cellular damage in the body. They could completely reverse the aging process as simply as changing graphics on a computer screen.

We know that this powerful, sub-Lilliputian technology is possible because the inspiration for it comes from nature. All living things are already built by biological molecular assemblers. This is simply the most precise way to build (or rebuild) material forms, as well as the cheapest and the fastest. Nanotechnology expert Eric Drexler says that this microscopic technology is inevitable given our present line of technological development in microelectronics, computers, and genetic engineering.

Through advances in computer science, software design, and the reverse engineering of the human brain, Kurzweil predicts that computer intelligence will exceed human intelligence in just a few decades and that it won't be long after that when humans start merging with machines, blurring the line between technology and biology.

Robotics expert Hans Moravec envisions Bush robots that will be able to repair virtually any type of damage to the human body. A Bush robot, according to Moravec, "is a branched hierarchy of articulated limbs, starting from a macroscopically large trunk through successively smaller and more numerous branches, ultimately leading to microscopic twigs and nanoscale fingers." This would make virtually any type of medical procedure possible as "even the most complicated procedures could be completed by a trillion-fingered robot, able, if necessary, to simultaneously work on almost every cell of a human body."

Through the combination of nanotechnology, advanced robotics, and escalating artificial intelligence, virtually anything that we can imagine really does become possible, and this is the subject of the next chapter. So it's true, for the first time in human history, that we really do stand on the brink of a miraculous New Age. Likewise, for the first time in human history we are perilously close to engineering our own extinction.

But again we must remind ourselves that it has always seemed this way to some people. Perhaps this is because the human adventure is simply an expression of deeper forces that are present at every level of organization in our universe—simultaneously driving the cosmos toward both higher order and more pronounced chaos.

Through the eons the whole evolution of life and technology that percolates up from the primordial oceans and into the heavens is locked in a constant battle against the forces of decay and the Second Law of Thermodynamics, which states that all systems that exchange energy are winding down into a state of entropy or disorder. One force always seems ready to devour the other, yet somehow they have remained in balance for around 15 billion years. Perhaps this is because these forces are ultimately part of larger whole, as the Chinese philosophy of Taoism would say.

However there does seem to be an escalation in the intensity of these two driving forces in the realm of human history, and the rate of cultural change appears to be ever accelerating. The dark seems to keep on getting darker, while the light appears to be getting brighter. Because of this apparent escalation, many people believe that we are headed toward a final showdown and that one of these forces—chaos or order—will finally prevail.

But I think this perspective comes from a limited view of the situation, and the coming of the end of the world and the dawn of the Great Awakening are both really just ever-persistent states of mind. I think the world will always appear this way from certain perspectives because of the way the universe is mysteriously constructed out of emptiness and radiance.

In reality the light and the dark elements of the world are always perfectly balanced, like the yin and yang of Taoism, although the balance appears to shift from our personal and collective experience, our emotions, our beliefs, our cultural imprinting, and the ever-changing state of the world at large. This is because we live in a dualistic universe where the creation of any cognitive distinction immediately creates its opposite. You can't have light without darkness to define it, and then complex layers upon layers of dark/light configuration patterns, which determine how we perceive the world, build up, congeal, and crystalize around one's most basic core beliefs about our perspective on the inherent good or bad nature of the world.

It seems to me that a basic trust in the greater life process in general is essential to our survival as individuals as well as the future evolution of our species. The biosphere, which has gotten us this far, is undoubtedly far wiser than we are, and this gives great reason to trust the process. Tapping in to this greater intelligence through my use of psychedelics gives me an even greater cause for optimism. I definitely get the feeling that the higher biospheric intelligence really knows what it's doing and has seen all of our current, seemingly insurmountable problems a billion trillion times before, and it is currently dealing with it accordingly (this book is an example). But, ultimately, I think our fate lies in our own hands.

As the game of life evolves the stakes just keep growing higher and higher. Computer games mimic this natural process in the universe, which forces us to encounter greater and greater challenges as our skills improve. I have yet to meet a person who says that life is a breeze. It challenges everyone to their core.

Is this toxic or nutritious? Is this shit or Shinola? We ask ourselves these questions about everything we encounter in every moment, and the choices we make guide our path through life—although nothing is really anything unless we believe it to be so, and our contexts continually shift the appearance of what is what. Of course, to make it all the more complicated, ultimately everything is composed of both dark and light forces, so it's wise for us to try to choose as carefully as possible.

With regard to our collective Self, we've never before had the power to destroy the whole biosphere or achieve immortality. Wow—aren't we something? We might think we're pretty tough now because we can blow up our own womb planet, but what happens when we gain the power to destroy stars, galaxies, or even universes?

A hundred years from now, if we keep evolving we'll develop enormous new powers and meet new challenges. We could destroy the whole galaxy by accident or malicious intent. I think that many species throughout the universe have already solved all of these problems long ago, and this suspicion or intuition deeply inspires me. If we do continue to grow, develop, and spiritually evolve, we could evolve into something beyond our wildest imaginings. Besides psychedelic mind states, another way to get in touch with what may lie beyond our wildest imagination is through lucid dreaming, which we'll be discussing more in the next chapter.

So with the highest potential of the imagination at our disposal, where are we heading? I think we're headed directly into our imagination.

DO CLUES TO OUR FUTURE EVOLUTION LIE IN OUR PAST?

The human species is continually evolving, and I suspect we're currently just an immature, larval form of what we are to become. We're like caterpillars who have yet to evolve into butterflies, as Leary surmised. But evolution may not always progress in a straight line, and the sobering truth is that most species on this planet are failed experiments that become extinct. But even in these cases, from a genetic/evolutionary perspective it's as if we're saying, "Oh, well. Let's try again and improve this new aspect of it." I suspect that evolution is intelligent, purposeful, and has an elaborate agenda in mind.

Ten thousand years ago on the southern tip of Africa there lived a species of humanlike primates who were about our size in height, only their heads were much larger and their faces were much smaller. They possessed brains that were around 30 to 35 percent larger than human brains, with a frontal cortex approximately 55 percent larger, and faces that were around one-fifth smaller. They were more highly evolved than us in the sense that compared to us, they were more neotenous.

The term *neoteny* refers to the mechanism in evolution whereby a new organism evolves from an existing species by retaining juvenile or larval characteristics into adulthood. The result is a sexually mature organism with a juvenile appearance that goes on to become a new species. Neoteny—also known as pedomorphosis—can be seen in many animals, and it is a common occurrence in the domestication of animals as pets. This is why, for example, dogs resemble juvenile wolves. According to evolutionary biologists, vertebrates evolved in this way from invertebrates, and amphibians in this manner from fish.

Humans tend to resemble young, relatively hairless apes. With this evolutionary trend in mind, isn't it interesting that many of the descriptions of extraterrestrials—in both the alien-abduction phenomenon and in science-fiction films—often resemble young human children or even human embryos?

Advanced extraterrestrials are often envisioned in science fiction and reported in alien encounters as having unusually large heads, big eyes, rudimentary noses, and small faces. These descriptions sound almost as if they could be an intuition about ourselves in the future—or, perhaps, a memory from our past. The faces of these creatures bare an uncanny resemblance to those of a species that has already evolved and perished (or vanished) on this planet. We have abundant fossil evidence that almost exactly this type of advanced primate lived in a region in South Africa known as Boskop between thirty thousand and ten thousand years ago.

The Boskops, or *Homo capensis* as they are known in anthropology, had much bigger brains than we do and were less apelike than we are. According to neuroscientists Gary Lynch and Richard Granger in their book *Big Brain,* the Boskops likely had cognitive abilities that far outperformed our own. They probably had much greater intelligence than we do, and because their frontal cortex was so large, they were also probably smarter than us in precisely those areas that we generally consider unique to human beings.

Boskops probably had a highly developed language, more advanced intellectual abilities, and a more sophisticated imagination. Their potential for science and art must have been staggeringly enormous, and one can only wonder what kind of spectacular mental abilities their superior brains were capable of. They must have been capable of having extraordinary psychedelic experiences that are beyond our wildest imaginings.

Physically the Boskops looked very different from us. An adult human face covers three-fifths of the head. The Boskop, with its large cranium, had a face with very large eyes that covered only two-fifths of its head, much like that of a three- or four-year-old human child.

Although the Boskops were probably much more intelligent than the human species, they're gone and no one knows what happened to them. They are considered a scientific anomaly, like crop circles, Bigfoot sightings, and psychic phenomena, and are rarely discussed by anthropologists. Did savage humans—our barbaric ancestors—slaughter their more peaceful, big-brained, doe-eyed cousins? Or did these superbrained geniuses evolve beyond us and just take off and leave? I like to think that they escaped into outer space or a higher dimension, but I realize that the more likely explanation is that we drove them to extinction.

Wherever they are, I miss them. I wish we had them here to help guide us through our present planetary crisis. I wish I had been able to interview a member of the species for one of my books, because archaeological evidence discussed by Lynch and Granger suggests that at least some ancient human societies regarded Boskops with great respect and sought them out for important matters of guidance. Their absence, perhaps, serves as a warning. Our civilization is much more fragile than it often appears, and we might not be as smart as we think, so these are crucial times where integrated intelligence and new ideas are greatly needed.

PAYING ATTENTION TO YOUTH CULTURE

Perhaps we can learn about the future evolution of our species by paying more attention to children, because they literally are the future.

When I asked media theorist Douglas Rushkoff what he thought adults can learn from youth culture, he replied:

> Why, they can learn about the future. Everybody tries to forecast the future using all sorts of strange methodologies about what's going to happen. So much effort has been expended exploring the question Where's the human race going? When all that you have to do is look at a kid. A kid is basically the next model of human being.

So if you want to know where evolution is taking us—whether it's physical evolution or cultural evolution—you look at kids, because they are quite literally the future.

Timothy Leary often spoke of humanity being at a larval stage in its development, with humans being analogous to caterpillars that have not yet evolved into butterflies. Leary pointed out that most animal species on this planet live in either the ocean or the air. If there is any type of teleology—design or intelligence—inherent in the evolutionary process, it would seem that gravity-bound creatures might be a transitional stage in evolution. Leary suggested that the human species might evolve into many thousands (or more) of new post-terrestrial, or postlarval, species as different as the various mammals or insects of today are from one another.

Certainly when we consider our evolutionary history a quick survey of our situation on this planet does seem to indicate that our species is at some sort of evolutionary crossroads. Could humans be the common ancestor to a vast array of future species, more varied in their form and abilities than the superpowered mutants in the *X-Men* movies? Could we be on the verge of branching off into a diverse extraterrestrial zoology that lives beyond the horizon of our imagination? Our wayward species may indeed be headed toward extinction, but maybe our descendants will evolve into something that does survive.

Perhaps the dinosaurs provide a compelling metaphor for the human species. No one is completely sure what killed off these massive, small-brained reptiles who ruled the Earth for 125 million years, as some evidence indicates that dinosaur populations began dwindling before the mass extinction occurred 65 million years ago. But when you think about the big picture from DNA's point of view, what really happened? The dinosaurs—these extremely large, cumbersome creatures whose genetics favored size and vicious violence over intelligence—were, over time and evolution, replaced by mammals and smaller, smarter, more mobile creatures who spend their days singing and soaring in the sky.

In other words, the smarter dinosaurs didn't die; they grew wings and evolved into what are today their only living descendants: birds. There may be a message here for human beings. Could we currently be facing an evolutionary crossroads similar to the one the dinosaurs faced 65 million years ago?

Douglas Rushkoff told me that the larger a multinational corporation grows, the smaller its brain becomes by comparison and the less control it has over what it's doing. Like the dinosaurs, part of us—the military-industrial complex, for example—may have grown disproportionately huge at the expense of other parts.

The challenge we are currently facing is because of an imbalance that comes from within ourselves, like with the dinosaurs. With the exception of natural disasters like earthquakes, hurricanes, and possibly asteroids, every problem that the human race is currently facing is entirely self-created. All that we really need to do in order to survive is learn how to get along with each other. If we can just learn to live together without killing each other, and be careful not to trash the environment, the human species will pass through a golden threshold into an age of miracles. But, apparently, this isn't as simple as it sounds.

This is why when science-fiction writers envision intelligent extraterrestrial civilizations they tend to equate advanced technology with advanced social and spiritual development. There just doesn't seem to be any other way to survive. The escalating dangers of combining high technology with violence and greed on our own planet make it clear that the potential for a global-scale disaster dramatically increases as a technologically sophisticated species matures. Unless a species' social and political capacities evolve with its technological advances and the members of the species learn how to get along with each other and their biosphere, it appears likely to destroy itself.

In his book *Critical Path,* the late Buckminster Fuller calculated that if the human race redirected all the money that is currently being spent on military budgets around the world, there would be enough resources on this planet for each person to live the lifestyle of a multimillionaire.

Just think of how utterly ridiculous our species would appear to an advanced extraterrestrial if we take this fact into account. If our planet's resources were redirected—away from what Robert Anton Wilson calls the death sciences (where the goal is to develop "faster and faster ways to kill more and more people") and into the life sciences (where the goal is to improve the quality of human life)—we could be living in a world that is truly limited only by the boundaries of our imaginations.

In the next chapter we'll be discussing the possibilities of pursuing promising avenues in the life sciences. But first let us ask ourselves, Just what would an extraterrestrial species think about what's happening on our wayward planet?

HAVE WE ALREADY BEEN VISITED BY EXTRATERRESTRIALS?

As anyone who has spoken with my mom will tell you, I've looked up into the night sky since I was a small child and wondered about the existence of extraterrestrial life. With every new discovery of yet another Earth-like planet in astrophysics, I become more and more convinced that our universe is simply seething with intelligent life, and I've always been fascinated, although not convinced, by archaeological finds that suggest possible human-alien contact in our past.

According to Superstring theorist Michio Kaku, one of my favorite authors on the subject of frontier physics, if highly advanced civilizations already visited us we may not even have had the ability to notice—that is, unless they wanted us to notice—as their probes could be so ultratiny and so carefully cloaked.

The late psychiatrist John Mack, author of the book *Abduction*, really perked my interest in this subject by suggesting that many people in our own time have had genuine contact experiences with intelligent nonhuman beings who appeared to come from somewhere far away from our world.

Like Timothy Leary, John was almost fired from his academic post at Harvard University for his unorthodox beliefs. I spoke with John at length about the alien-abduction phenomenon, and I interviewed him several times. John presents an abundance of compelling evidence to show that many people have had experiences where they genuinely believe they were abducted by extraterrestrials, and they report many similar details. The conversations I had with John were condensed in my book *Conversations on the Edge of the Apocalypse*. I find this subject utterly fascinating, although I'm not quite sure what to make of it. There really are some extremely compelling reasons to take these reports seriously, which become apparent after one carefully examines the literature.

When I interviewed DMT researcher Rick Strassman he told me he thought the alien-abduction phenomenon was because of elevated DMT levels in the brain. There are certainly a lot of similarities between the experiences to support this idea. Many DMT voyagers reported being helpless in the presence of advanced aliens in a hospital or laboratory setting or being given some kind of medical procedure, which is reminiscent of many alien-abduction reports. (I'll be discussing this much more in the next chapter.) When I asked Rick about this he said:

> I think that, based upon what many of our volunteers experienced viz entity contact, high levels of DMT could break down the subjective/objective membrane separating us from other levels of reality, in which perhaps some of these entities "reside." I've been criticized by the abduction community because of the lack of objective evidence of encounters in our volunteers—e.g., stigmata, metal objects, etc. In response to these concerns, it might be worth considering a spectrum of encounters—from the purely material (about which I withhold all judgment), to the purely consciousness-to-consciousness contact experience that may usefully describe what our volunteers underwent.

When I interviewed John Mack about the connection between psychedelic experiences and the alien-abduction phenomenon he said:

I find that interesting. It's very mysterious. I've seen this too, and it does seem that when some people take psychedelics they may open themselves up to something that seems similar. Terence McKenna talks about taking DMT and then suddenly finding all kinds of alien beings around him. What does this mean? Obviously it didn't cause something to materialize physically, so it suggests that, in a certain sense, the person has become proactive in discovering another realm. Those cases may be experienced quite similarly to the cases where there's actual physical evidence that some material UFO has actually appeared in somebody's backyard, but that doesn't help me with the situation I face. I have cases where a neighbor or the media report a UFO close to somebody's home, or where they were driving their car, and independently the person will tell me about a UFO abduction experience. They don't know that the media has tracked the UFO.

So there is a physical dimension to this. And it's that aspect of it that has created so much distress in Western culture, because we felt we were safely cornered off in our material sanctity. The idea that some kind of entities, beings, or energies from some other dimension can cross over and find us here, in a way that no missile-defense is going to help, is scary to most people. It doesn't scare me particularly. But I guess that's scary if you've been raised with the notion that we're the preeminent bosses of the cosmos and nobody can get us, and all we have to do is create better technologically controlled atmospheres, astrodomes, and that kind of thing, and no one will ever reach us. I mean, think about what the military's Star Wars project is. The Strategic Defense Initiative is based on the belief that somehow technology can make us secure and inviolate from ourselves and the powers and energies of the cosmos. I've read most of Terence McKenna's books, and I find they're very compatible with what I'm about. But I don't think he quite realizes how robust the abduction phenomenon itself is, because his access to it has been so much through psychedelics. I don't think he realizes how powerful these crossover experiences are in a material sense.

So John thought there was more of a physical dimension to these types of encounters than just journeys of the soul into hyperspace. This is one of those areas where there is strangely compelling evidence, if one delves into it deeply, enough to convince any reasonably minded person that something mysterious is going on, but without enough evidence to convince a hard-nosed skeptic. I suspect that these types of experiences are evidence for a mischievous presence among us that I like to call daimons.

MISCHIEVOUS DAIMONIC SPIRITS IN OUR MIDST

John Mack introduced me to a book by Patrick Harpur called *Daimonic Reality,* which changed my view on a lot of unexplained phenomena. I've always been fascinated by anomalies that can't quite be explained by science—something that Rupert Sheldrake taught me to be keenly observant of when we worked together. Harpur's book pooled a number of commonly known, unexplained phenomena that had strongly compelling evidence to support the claims, yet never quite the definitive proof to convince a hard-core skeptic. When presented together in such detail it almost seems like some kind of higher intelligence is toying with us to produce Bigfoot sightings, crop circles, alien abductions, and other strange phenomena reported by reliable witnesses that defy conventional scientific explanations.

Harpur presents the intriguing view that the reason aliens appear to us in the so-called abduction phenomenon as technologically superadvanced, sterile, cold, scientific beings merely interested in our medical nature are, in effect, parodying us. According to Harpur they're mocking us by coming in a form that we would imagine our future to be like and how we know our species treats other animals in our laboratories. They're making fun of us to teach us an important lesson about where we're going. I like this idea, and it rings true with a friend's DMT encounter of technologically advanced monkeys wearing sunglasses, and the powerful ketamine experience I'll be describing in the next chapter, where the extraterrestrial scientists who were experimenting on me during the experience appeared as giant rabbits.

4

Approaching the Singularity

As I discussed in the previous chapter, despite all the escalating chaos, confusion, and ever-increasing darkness easily observed in the world today, I am now more optimistic than ever before about the future evolution of our species. No matter where one turns for evidence, I'm convinced that an infinite amount of data will become available to support his or her point of view, but I've deliberately chosen to take an optimistic perspective because it seems more likely to generate a more positive outcome for me and the world.

When I interviewed technology expert Ray Kurzweil he described how our technological progress is inevitably leading us into a world that is beyond our wildest imagination. According to Kurzweil, who has a stellar track record of predicting technological advances, our technological developments are advancing at an exponential rate and it won't be long before human intelligence becomes indistinguishable from artificial intelligence.

Then, according to Kurzweil, it won't be long after that our computers become more intelligent than we are, merging with us in the process and carrying us along into what he refers to as the Singularity. This term, which I mentioned earlier, is borrowed from physics, and it describes a place where the known laws of physics break down, like inside a collapsed star, and future predictions become impossible because entirely new variables come into play.

One of the first things that one notices about Kurzweil is how young and healthy he looks for a man of sixty-four. While it's likely that Kurzweil takes more nutritional supplements than anyone else on Earth, and he certainly takes excellent care of his health, his optimism may also be a contributing factor to his youthful appearance. Scientific studies have demonstrated that optimistic people live longer than pessimistic people. Robert Anton Wilson made this point a lot, and he and Timothy Leary deeply inspired me with their boundless sense of optimism. In a world plagued by so much fear and pessimism, I vowed to try my best to do the same—and have been very happy with the results so far.

NEOPHOBIA AND NEOPHILIA

I've noticed for a long time that children and young people tend to be more optimistic than older adults, and there also tends to be more cultural optimism in the West than the East, where societies are older and more conservative. I've wondered for a long time about why this seems to be so. Older people who are more pessimistic tell me that they're simply more realistic, but my younger friends have convinced me otherwise, and I've thought that there is a tendency for neophobia to increase with age, especially if one doesn't do psychedelics or travel much to other cultures.

When I was studying psychobiology as an undergraduate at the University of Southern California in 1981 one of my research projects involved the study of neophobia, or the fear of novelty. My research involved measuring the interspatial distance between identical schools of fish, in both familiar and novel environments, to see if there was any difference. In my study I found that the fish tended to school closer together in novel environments. Not exactly the most exciting discovery, I'll admit, but I also learned much more about neophobia by studying the research of others. I was fascinated to discover that in all studied organisms neophobia does indeed tend to increase with age. Older animals tend to be more suspicious and distrustful of environmental changes than young animals.

It soon became clear to me that this is also an obvious pattern in human beings. Young people tend to be more idealistic, curious, and optimistic—more neophilic (novelty loving); older people tend to be more suspicious and pessimistic—more neophobic (novelty fearing). Both forces, it seems, are necessary for advancing evolution. Part of the reason why I'm so optimistic, I think, is because of my copious use of psychedelic drugs, which has tended to keep my perspective fresh and my mind young, that is, neotenous. Young minds tend to be more open to novelty than older minds. According to Terence McKenna we're descending to a point of infinite novelty. So if he's right, I think that it's probably wise to be as prepared as possible.

THE CAMBRIAN EXPLOSION AND THE SINGULARITY

Life has been evolving on Earth for a few billion years, and, as we discussed in the first chapter, the earliest fossil records show that human beings first appeared on the scene around a hundred million or two hundred million years ago. Then, around forty thousand years ago, there was a dramatic, planetary-wide progression of human culture that anthropologists are scratching their heads trying to account for.

Some people have suggested the possibility of some kind of intervention by an advanced species of extraterrestrials, but this wasn't the first time in the history of life on this planet that there was such a big, unexplained development. During what is known as the Cambrian explosion, which took place around 530 million years ago, there was a relatively rapid appearance of many new species, accompanied by a major diversification of other organisms. Before about 580 million years ago most organisms were relatively simple, composed only of individual cells that occasionally organized into colonies. During the Cambrian explosion, which occurred over a period of 70 million or 80 million years, the rate of evolution accelerated at an unprecedented magnitude.

The late biologist Stephen Jay Gould has suggested that evolution doesn't generally progress in the gradual manner that many evolutionary biologists think, but rather long periods of relative stability are punctuated by periods of rapid evolutionary advancement. I personally suspect that this process is guided by ancient, superwise, genetic-biospheric intelligence that is itself further aligned with the greater purpose of the intelligence of the cosmos. But what do I know? No more than you. Whatever the case, it appears that evolution is an ever-accelerating process, and we can only guess what lies over the edge of the horizon.

When I do my best to envision what entering the Singularity or descending into infinite novelty might actually be like, I naturally recall those experiences where I personally encountered the most novelty at once. These times unquestionably occurred during the experiments that I did on myself with N,N-dimethyltryptamine (DMT).

THE MYSTERY OF DMT

One of the most mysterious puzzles in all of nature—in the same league as questions like "What existed before the Big Bang?" "How did life begin?" and "Why am I here?"—revolves around the fact that the unusually powerful psychedelic DMT is naturally found in the human body as well as in many species of animals and plants, and no biochemist can tell you what it does in any of these places. After talking with a number of expert neuroscientists and biochemists on this subject I had to conclude that nobody really has the slightest idea why DMT is found naturally in our bodies and all throughout nature. However, it's mysterious and ubiquitous presence appears to be a message of some sort.

Because natural DMT levels tend to rise while we're asleep at night, a biochemical role in dreaming has been suggested by some neuroscientists. However this is entirely speculation, and even if this is true it may also do more. DMT is one of the primary ingredients in ayahuasca, the potent hallucinogenic jungle juice from the Amazon, and because of its endogenous status and unusually potent effects many people have considered it to be the quintessential psychedelic.

I agree. Personally, I think that all of the psychedelic experiences that are made possible with the multitude of new synthetic designer psychedelics are merely subsets of what is possible with the ayahuasca experience. I suspect that ayahuasca is the mother of all psychedelic experiences.

DMT has effects of such strength and magnitude that it easily dwarfs the titanic quality of even the most powerful LSD trips, and it appears to transport one into an entirely new world—a world that seems more bizarre than our wildest imaginings yet somehow is also strangely familiar.

Psychiatric researcher Rick Strassman, who conducted a five-year study with DMT at the University of New Mexico between 1990 and 1995, has suggested that naturally elevated DMT levels in the brain may be responsible for such unexplained mental phenomena as spontaneous religious experiences, near-death experiences, nonhuman entity contact, and psychosis. Strassman—who suspects that DMT is likely produced in the pineal gland—and others have even gone so far as to speculate about the possibility that elevated DMT levels in the brain might be responsible for ushering the soul into the body before we're born and out of the body after its demise.

However, what's most interesting about DMT is that, with great consistency, it appears to allow human beings to communicate with other intelligent life-forms.

NONHUMAN ENTITY CONTACT

When I interviewed Strassman I asked him if he thought there was any objective reality to the strange worlds visited by people when they're under the influence of DMT and if he thought that the entities so many people have encountered there actually have a genuine, independent existence. Rick replied:

> I myself think so. My colleagues think I've gone woolly-brained over this, but I think it's as good a working hypothesis as any other. I tried all other hypotheses with our volunteers, and with myself. The "this is your brain on drugs" model; the Freudian "this is your unconscious playing out repressed wishes and fears"; the Jungian "these are archetypal images symbolizing your unmet potential"; the "this is a dream"; etc. Volunteers had powerful objections to all of these explanatory models—and they were a very sophisticated group of volunteers, with decades of psychotherapy, spiritual practice, and previous psychedelic experiences. I tried a thought-experiment, asking myself, "What if these were real worlds, and real entities? Where would they reside, and why would they care to interact with us?" This led me to some interesting speculations about parallel universes, dark matter, etc. All because we can't prove these ideas right now (lacking the proper technology) doesn't mean they should be dismissed out of hand as incorrect.

I asked Terence McKenna what he thought about this and how—in these profoundly powerful psychedelic states—he was able to distinguish between independently operating parts of himself and other intelligences. He responded by saying:

> It's very hard to differentiate it. How can I make that same distinction right now? How do I know I'm talking to you? It's just provisionally assumed, that you are ordinary enough that I don't question that you're there. But if you had two heads, I would question whether you were there. I would investigate to see if you were really what you appear to be. It's very hard to tell what this I/thou relationship is about, because it's very difficult to define the "I" part

of it, let alone the "thou" part of it. I haven't found a way to tell, to trick it as it were into showing whether it was an extraterrestrial or the back side of my own head . . . this is simply a voice . . . so it's the issue of the mysterious telephone call. If you're awakened in the middle of the night by a telephone call, and you pick up the phone, and someone says "Hello" it would not be your first inclination to ask "Is anybody there?" because they just said hello. That establishes that somebody is there. But you can't see them, so maybe they aren't there. Maybe you've been called by a machine. I've been called by machines. You pick up the phone and it says, "Hello this is Sears, and we're calling to tell you that your order 16312 is ready for pick up." And you say, "Oh, thank you." "Don't mention it." No, so this issue of identifying the other with certainty is tricky, even in ordinary intercourse.

When I spoke with Rupert Sheldrake I asked him whether he thought that the DMT entities might be able to sense that they are being stared at. Sheldrake told me that he thinks people can sense that they are being stared at, because when we are looking at someone a part of the observer is, in a sense, actually reaching out to touch the person being observed in some way. I was curious as to whether he thought this was true in other states of consciousness, where the person one is observing is not in consensus material reality. For example, in lucid dreams, DMT-induced states of consciousness, or in a computer-simulated virtual reality, did he think that the act of looking at someone—or some being—in one of these alternative realities is actually expanding a part of that person's mind into another dimension of sorts, or did he think this might be an illusion that's just in the mind? When I asked him about this he replied:

I think these things are in the mind, but I don't think the mind is in the brain. I think in an ordinary act of vision, when we look at something, the mind extends beyond our brain. If I look out of my window now and see a tree, I don't think that image of the tree is inside my head. I think the image is where it seems to be. I think it's projected out. Vision involves a two-way process. Light moving in, changes in the brain, and then projection out of images. And oddly enough, when you think about the conventional theory, that it's all in the brain, it leads to very peculiar consequences. I'm looking up at the sky now, and according to the conventional view, my image of the sky, what I'm seeing in front of me, is actually inside my head. That means that my skull must be beyond the sky. When you look up at the sky, your skull's beyond the sky. Now this is absurd really, and yet that's what the conventional view is telling us, and most people take it for granted, without realizing how very counterintuitive, and very peculiar this speculative theory is. So I think that we go beyond our brain in the simplest act of vision, and I think that many of these other experiences also involve going beyond the brain. I don't think the mind is confined to the brain. So it may be true to say that near-death experiences, visionary experiences, and DMT trips are all in the mind, but that doesn't mean to say they're all in the brain.

Computer scientist Marko A. Rodriguez published a scientific paper in 2008 called "A Methodology for Studying Various Interpretations of the N,N-dimethyltryptamine-Induced Alternate Reality" that explores how to possibly determine if the entities experienced by people under the influence of DMT are really independently existing, intelligent beings, or merely the projections of our chemically altered brains. Rodriguez suggests using a cognitive test that involves asking the entities to perform a complex mathematical task involving prime numbers in order to verify their independent existence. While it seems like quite a long shot that this method will lead to any kind of fruitful results, I think any serious speculation about establishing communication channels with these mysterious beings can be constructive.

Smoking, injecting, or snorting DMT in a purified form can be extremely intense and highly stimulating, beyond overwhelming at the higher dosages, and this is how it earned the underground nickname DPT, which stands for double-penetration tryptamine. Doing DMT can sometimes be extremely frightening. The heightened state of anxiety that sometimes occurs with high-dose levels of DMT, according to McKenna, stems from the "fear that one will die of astonishment . . . and is a hallmark of the experience's authenticity."

Anyone who has read Rick Strassman's marvelous book *DMT: The Spirit Molecule* was probably struck by the report of how one of Strassman's test subjects terrifyingly believed that he was being anally raped by a monster alligator during his DMT experience. I wonder what Terence would have said to this person. In any case, I discovered this mother of all fears firsthand the very first time I tried DMT.

DJB MEETS DMT

I first tried smoking DMT in 1983, when I was twenty-one years old. I was at the home of a friend named Bruce, who offered to introduce me to the experience, which I had read about and had wanted to try for years. I blessed his heart as he scraped together some loose orange-red crystals from the bottom of a kitchen drawer and carefully placed them into the bottom of a huge glass pipe in his living room. Then I sat down on the couch as he fired up the bowl of the pipe from the bottom with a strong blowtorch lighter and vaporized the DMT crystals, while I inhaled three deep lungfuls of the vapor. This was to become the most powerful psychedelic experience of my life.

The vapor tasted like burned plastic and felt horrible in my lungs, like molten glass scorching the inside of my chest. Within seconds after smoking the first lungful of the DMT I felt like I was peaking on the highest LSD trip I'd ever been on. The absolutely insane kaleidoscopic patterns that were unfolding before me were an order of magnitude more intense than anything I had previously witnessed on LSD, mescaline, or psilocybin. Somehow I managed to inhale two more lungfuls of the awful-tasting vapor, and a few seconds later I found myself in a completely different, higher-ordered dimension, complex beyond anything I can adequately describe in human language.

It was impossible to gain my orientation during the experience, and I witnessed the most incredible things imaginable. This was not a human world that I was in; it was populated by other intelligent creatures, and I was able to see my ever-morphing environment—their world—in 360 degrees. So much was going on around me. I watched in spellbound fascination as legions of small, elflike beings were diving into this strange biological machine and sliding out of it, like it was an amusement-park ride. It appeared to be giving them enormous pleasure to do this. (Years later, through subsequent experiences with DMT, I began to suspect that this "amusement-park ride" was actually the entrance into a three-dimensional human body where one experienced a lifetime, which seemed like just a brief moment from the perspective of hyperspace. I heard about someone's experience with an extract made from the African iboga root that was similar, in which they found themselves in a postdeath realm with access to a "reincarnation machine," and beings could experience whole human lifetimes virtually instantaneously from the perspective of that realm.)

Suddenly I felt myself in the grip of an intelligent being that was doing something to me that I didn't understand. I kept trying to interpret what the being was and what was happening and felt utterly helpless. I projected what seemed like millions of possible interpretations per second onto this complex being, but nothing in my mind fit or seemed to make sense. I alternated between states of ecstatic pleasure and absolute terror as I wondered, *Is this being a scientist experimenting on me? Is "he" good or bad? Is this being someone that I already know somehow? Is "he" a friend? A lover? A parent? An angel? A demon? An extraterrestrial? Is it God, or my own creator?*

In some weird way it seemed that this being was a giant version of myself, a gigantically huge and all-powerful "David Jay Brown," that was measuring and adjusting reactions in my brain with extreme precision, as "he" administered a vast series of intensifying stimuli that seemed to be activating all of my senses at once to their maximum thresholds. Energies poured into me, beyond my capacity to handle, as this being adjusted the range of streaming sensations, twisting (what seemed like) different-colored light filters over me, asking me repeatedly, with each click or change: "Like this?" It seemed like "he" was trying to determine when the intensity of the sensations would become too much for me, in one brain area or perceptual range after another, while I was desperately trying to understand what in the world was happening.

This towering being seemed to be measuring and adjusting different threshold sensitivities in my brain for experiencing pleasure and pain. I vividly remember how strong sweet and bitter, sometimes metallic, taste sensations strangely and synesthetically blended with continuously transforming extradimensional visual imagery as I pleaded with the being to please stop. I learned later from Bruce that I actually said these words out loud during the experience, while I was being experimented on in another dimension. It was simply too much for my poor little monkey brain to handle, and much of what happened that afternoon is impossible to remember.

When I started to come back to Earth it took me what felt like forever just to remember that I was a human being who had done a drug. Although it felt like an eternity, only around ten minutes had actually gone by before I was back in my body, asking Bruce how long it had been. I sat there saying "Wow" over and over as I watched a powerful and vividly colorful tapestry of bejeweled patterns fluidly unfold, morph, and merge, ultimately solidifying into the walls and furniture of Bruce's apartment. For around ten more minutes I felt like I was being shown secrets about how everything in our reality was constructed behind the scenes, so to speak, much like on a high-dose magic mushroom trip.

I was back to baseline in thirty minutes after smoking the DMT. This experience became the basis for a scene in the second chapter of my first science-fiction novel, *Brainchild*. Many of the scenes in my science-fiction novels came directly from my trip reports, and like Philip K. Dick and Robert Anton Wilson, I sometimes had difficulty distinguishing my science fiction from reality.

Encountering that strange being on my first DMT trip wasn't the only time that I felt like an extraterrestrial scientist was experimenting on my brain.

KETAMINE AND MY ENCOUNTER WITH THE EXTRATERRESTRIAL RABBIT SCIENTISTS

When I was in graduate school at the University of Southern California, studying behavioral neuroscience at the Hedco Neurosciences Center, the research I was involved in required that I surgically implant cold probes into the brains (the cerebellar cortex, specifically) of rabbits. This was precisely the opposite of the research that I did at NYU, where we used electrodes to stimulate specific regions of the brain; cold probes temporarily freeze and deactivate specific brain regions.

When I was at NYU I did research where I surgically implanted electrical brain-stimulation electrodes into the lateral hypothalamus of Sprague Dawley rats, which is an important pleasure/reward center. This was a continuation of the earlier research that John Lilly pioneered at the National Institutes of Health in the 1950s. I would sit in the lab for hours, watching the single-minded rats press a bar that delivered an electric current into their brain's reward center over and over again until, eventually, they dropped from exhaustion. Then, a few hours later, they would wake up and start doing it all over again.

There was food sitting next to them, water sitting next to them, and a fertile mate sitting next to them; they ignored all three and would continue to press that bar over and over again to get the rewarding electrical stimulation, in spite of their survival instincts. Although I never experimented on myself with electrical brain stimulation, I fantasized about doing it—and these fantasies became the foundation for my novel *Brainchild*.

When I was working in the USC neuroscience labs in 1989, the drug that we used to anesthetize our furry experimental subjects (Dutch-belted rabbits) prior to surgery was an anesthetic called ketamine. I knew from having read John Lilly's books that ketamine was also a powerful hallucinogen. I had read about how John had used ketamine to travel out of his body and make contact with extraterrestrial intelligences.

I wanted to try ketamine for myself, and this seemed to be considerably safer than implanting electrodes in my brain. I was, however, later to discover that the same type of addictive behavior that I witnessed with the rats pressing bars to deliver an electric current over and over into their brain, at the expense of all else, was indeed quite similar to the seductive loops that many people got caught up in with ketamine, including John Lilly and, for a time, me. I've watched many people mechanically inject ketamine into themselves over and over until their supply runs out. There was a strange irony in watching John Lilly do this with ketamine, injecting it over and over again, after he had pioneered the original self-stimulation, electrical brain-stimulation research with monkeys who had acted so similarly.

In any case, one evening I bravely took a bottle of ketamine home with me from the USC neuroscience lab along with a few sterile syringes. When I got home I settled onto my bed, wiped my leg with some rubbing alcohol, and safely injected 90 milligrams of ketamine into my right thigh muscle. Then I turned out the lights. Five minutes later I suddenly "realized" that my doctoral advisers at USC were really extraterrestrial scientists who had been videotaping me in the lab while I wasn't aware of it and were secretly watching and studying my every move. In fact they had actually left the bottle of ketamine for me to take, and they were watching me right at that moment.

I also "realized" that they weren't really interested in the neural mechanics of rabbit brains; that was just a disguise, and they were really experimenting on me. I was the real test subject. I suddenly found myself completely naked, inside of a locked cage, with cold probes stuck into my head. Giant rabbits were all around me, and they appeared to know everything that was going on in my mind. They were watching and measuring me right at that moment. I felt totally helpless, at their mercy, and the sole purpose of my life now seemed as though it was to fulfill some routine research function for these giant rabbit scientists.

Even though the trip only lasted for around forty-five minutes, after that experience I was never able to see the neuroscience lab and the research I was doing there in the same way again. I felt way too much empathy with the test subjects, although I did wonder what they experienced while on ketamine. Needless to say I didn't last much longer in that graduate program.

KETAMINE AND JOHN LILLY

However, I did continue to experiment with ketamine. I became good friends with John Lilly, and for about a year we regularly did ketamine together at his Malibu estate (while I was dating his beautiful adopted daughter, Barbara). My interview with John appears in my book *Mavericks of the Mind*. Ketamine is a difficult drug to categorize. Pharmacologically it's classified as a dissociative anesthetic, along with MXE, nitrous oxide, DXM, and PCP, as they all bind to the NMDA receptors in the brain, where they help to control synaptic plasticity and memory function. They all have somewhat similar subjective effects as well.

Unlike the classical psychedelics, ketamine and other dissociative anesthetics can be psychologically addicting (because of their accompanying opiate-like euphoria), and often what one experiences during the trip is difficult to remember. Emerging from a ketamine trip is like coming out of a dissolving dream. What was suddenly so intensely vivid just moments before now slips through your fingers like running water as you try to recall it. Nonetheless, powerful lasting insights and amazing out-of-body experiences can be had if one uses the drug wisely and respectfully. However, beware: I've encountered some strangely delusional thinking while on ketamine, like when I became convinced that my landlady had snuck into my apartment and switched my telephone for a different one. I almost called her about it during the trip to complain.

When I asked John how he thought ketamine should best be experienced in the isolation tank, he said:

> My major guideline when I go in the tank is, for God's sake don't preprogram, don't have a purpose, let it happen. With ketamine and LSD I did the same thing; I slowly let go of controlling the experience. You know some people lie in the tank for an hour trying to experience what I experienced. Finally, I wrote an introduction to *The Deep Self,* and said, if you really want to experience what it is to be in the tank, don't read any of my books, don't listen to me, just go in there and be.

Ketamine works in a pharmacological way that's precisely the opposite from classical psychedelics; rather than enhancing the senses, it closes them down. In higher doses there are uncanny similarities between where DMT and ketamine bring one to, and this is why the "party" doses of ketamine that people snort at dance clubs produce a euphoric dissociative buzz, but it's not usually terribly psychedelic. DMT seems to carry you up into these states of hyperspace, while ketamine seems to lower you down into them.

The best way that I found to do ketamine in a shamanic context was with 100-milligram doses by intramuscular injection, as its oral availability seems inconsistent and it's pretty difficult to snort enough ketamine to have the kind of experiences that John Lilly and I have described.

However, I've had success snorting the ketamine analog MXE, which has similar effects but is much more potent and longer lasting. The first time I tried this fascinating substance it felt like a three-hour ketamine trip where my mind floated in a gelatin matrix, telepathically intertwined with the mind of my lover, while other minds buzzed about us. With repeated use ketamine experiences become like lucid dreams, where one can interact with new worlds. The best places to do ketamine, John and I both agree, are inside an isolation tank, lying peacefully on a bed in the dark, or cuddling with a lover in bed with the lights out.

I had numerous really strange experiences with ketamine, after experimenting with it regularly for around a year in my early thirties. One night I did some ketamine with a girlfriend, and we were cuddling together in bed. I suddenly heard her voice in my head and began telepathically conversing with her. I was absolutely amazed that this was happening. We never vocalized a word, and I telepathically asked her several times to squeeze my hand, just to confirm that the telepathic conversations were indeed real.

Each time, several times, she confirmed it by squeezing my hand. We fell asleep in each other's arms, and when we awoke in the morning the first thing I said was that the previous night had been so incredibly amazing and that I had never experienced anything like that before. She asked me what I was referring to, and I said, "You know. The telepathic conversation that we had last night on ketamine," but she had no idea what I was talking about.

Another time I did ketamine with my girlfriend and suddenly found myself inside a huge, domed underwater arena where I was now occupying the body of a multi-tentacled alien creature making love to another multi-tentacled alien creature. This went on for a while until I suddenly snapped back in to my human body, which was in the process of making love to my girlfriend. The sudden shift between the different bodies and different worlds was jolting and totally freaked me out. I had to stop making love and just try to figure out what in the world was going on.

Every time I saw John his standard greeting was, "Got any K?" I would usually respond by saying, "I love you too, John."

For more information about ketamine I highly recommend John Lilly's book *The Scientist* and Karl Jansen's book *Ketamine: Dreams and Realities.*

AYAHUASCA AND THE FUTURE

Both ketamine and DMT can produce profound out-of-body experiences, but DMT appears to do so with a much greater range of emotion. During my ketamine experiences I felt completely transcendent of my emotions; however, with DMT one of the major obstacles that I had to overcome was primal fear.

I've smoked DMT numerous times since my first experience, usually in much smaller doses and often combined with LSD and harmaline, which made my experiences with DMT much more meaningful, manageable, and, dare I say, enjoyable. DMT and harmaline are truly a match made in heaven. Harmaline is an MAO-inhibiting enzyme that's found in a number of plants, like the famous South American vine *Banisteriopsis caapi,* which composes half of the mixture in the sacred hallucinogenic jungle juice ayahuasca. Harmaline is widely known as the chemical that allows the DMT in other plants, like *Psychotria viridis,* to become orally active.

Orally consumed DMT is destroyed in the stomach by an enzyme called monoamine oxidase (MAO), which harmaline inhibits. However, it does much more than just make the DMT orally active. I discovered that drinking a tea made from Syrian rue seeds two hours prior to smoking DMT dramatically alters the experience of smoking DMT. Harmaline has interesting psychoactive properties of its own that are somewhat psychedelic. I see colored trails following moving objects while on it. There's a cannabis-like mental buzz and a drunken, uncoordinated feeling in my muscles, along with a mild to moderate amount of nausea.

I also tend to feel as though I'm in touch with what I can only describe as Earth spirits—intelligent presences that seem to be trying to teach or show me things about the nature of spiritual development—while under the influence of harmaline. These spirits seem different from the strange extradimensional neuroscientists and hypercomplex insectoid beings that I've encountered while on pure DMT, as though the harmaline beings are more familiar and ancestral. They seem like the spirits of other creatures from our Earth's biosphere, part of the planetary family of biological beings from which we arose. It appears that these spirits are always around us and are always subtly communicating with us, but their changing ethereal forms are usually invisible and their presence is normally barely perceptible to our otherwise focused attention.

Smoking DMT two hours after drinking a couple of cups of Syrian rue tea is a completely different experience than smoking it on its own. It produces an experience much like that produced by ayahuasca, without much of the nausea that often comes from drinking the Amazonian jungle brew.

When I did this for the first time I noticed how much smoother and easier it was to inhale the usually harsh DMT vapors. It felt about as easy and comfortable as smoking cannabis. The next thing I noticed was that the trip began much more slowly. Instead of taking just a few seconds for the morphing kaleidoscopic patterns to start unfolding, it now took almost a full minute. The effects would usually begin just as I was exhaling the spent vapor, and then the experience would progress slower. The whole experience became stretched out over a longer period of time, around twice the duration or more, and I was able examine what was happening much more thoughtfully and carefully.

Every time I've smoked DMT while on harmaline I've begun to sense other intelligent presences around and within me, talking to me in English, explaining secrets about the nature of existence, healing and health, ecology and the biosphere, life and death, the genetic wiring of human beings, and the larger evolutionary plan in store for us. I've had "spirits" give me step-by-step instructions in English about how to properly massage a traveling companion who was suffering from physical discomforts during a shamanic journey, which seemed to work quite well. These Amazonian shamans aren't kidding around when they say that the plant spirits talk to them. Much of what I've been shown by these beings involved our evolutionary future, and this is where many of the ideas in my science-fiction novels came from.

I should clarify that when I refer to DMT, I mean the N,N variety, not the 5-MeO variety. These two chemical analogs have similar psychoactive effects, but the N,N variety produces far more visual imagery, and the 5-MeO variety is more potent, so less of it needs to be smoked for a strong effect. Most of my 5-MeO-DMT experiences have been largely disappointing as they felt like N,N-DMT mentally and physically, just with most of the astonishing morphing visual imagery starkly missing. However, James Oroc has convinced me of this substance's unique value in his book *Tryptamine Palace,* which describes how strong enough doses of 5-MeO-DMT can reliably produce powerful unions with what people can only describe as God. The most pleasant, visual, and emotionally powerful experience that I ever had with 5-MeO-DMT was when I tried combining it with a wonderful psilocybin mushroom extract and opium poppy tea, which was truly divine.

In any case, it's difficult for us as a species to understand what evolves after we do. For all of human history optimal health, longevity, freedom, art, science, and spirituality have been the goals or fruits. For the species that we're giving birth to, this is merely their starting point—that is, if we don't drive ourselves into extinction first and set the biosphere's development back a few hundred thousand years, which, from its perspective, is really nothing at all.

Our imagination, our dreams, intuitions, premonitions, and our psychedelic visions may give us a clue as to where we're headed.

THE REALITY OF LUCID DREAMING

A lucid dream is a dream where the dreamer is conscious of the fact that he or she is dreaming within a dream, while it happening. As a result, one is able to take an active role in the dream, where he or she becomes almost like a deity in the dream reality, imbued with the incredible omnipotent power to make just about anything happen.

Stanford University psychophysiologist Stephen LaBerge, whom I interviewed for my book *Mavericks of the Mind,* and who also appeared on one of the roundtable discussions that I cohosted, made the study of lucid dreaming into a science by demonstrating its undisputed reality. (That is, naively assuming, that this reality is undisputed.) LaBerge began researching lucid dreaming for his Ph.D. in psychophysiology at Stanford, which he received in 1980, and has done numerous studies on the subject since then. Although some people, largely philosophers, have been reporting lucid dream experiences throughout history—some advanced yogis routinely report whole nights of lucid dreaming— many dream researchers remained skeptical before LaBerge's conclusive studies.

The skeptical researchers claimed that people were only dreaming or imagining that they were lucid and they weren't truly conscious in the waking sense; they just remembered the dream as if they had been lucid. So LaBerge devised an unusually clever experiment to show that some people are every bit as conscious in a lucid dream as they are in what we call normal waking consciousness.

Here's what LaBerge did. He recruited a group of extremely sophisticated dreamers, or "psychonauts" as he affectionately called them— people with a seeming natural instinct for lucid dreaming who had trained themselves to become quite adept at maintaining lucidity in their dream states—and LaBerge taught them techniques for developing these skills even further. LaBerge had the subjects spend whole nights sleeping in his dream laboratory, where their brain waves and other physiological signals could be closely monitored.

Before the subjects went to sleep they and LaBerge agreed on a specific code of symbols to communicate from the dream state to the external world in order to demonstrate lucidity. When we fall asleep the physical body becomes mostly paralyzed so that the muscles we move in our dream body don't (thank goodness) move our actual physical limbs much—with one exception: our eye muscles. Eye movements in dreams precisely correspond to the eye movements of our physical bodies, and it appears that the rapid eye movements (REM) recorded in dream states actually reflect what we're looking at in our dreams.

So LaBerge instructed his subject to communicate with specially coordinated eye movements while in the lucid dream state. Once the subjects found themselves in a dream, which was externally confirmed by EEG (brain wave) monitoring, they then executed a preselected code of eye movements—such as two movements to the right, three to the left, four to the right, and one to the left, kind of like Morse code. These experiments produced significant results, demonstrating that people are able to remember that they are dreaming within a dream and are able to carry out a predetermined sequence of actions while in the dream.

Since these experiments, LaBerge has written several popular books on the subject, and he teaches workshops about lucid dreaming as a large interest in the subject has grown over the past two decades. LaBerge also developed a technological tool called the DreamLight, which helps people to lucid dream. The DreamLight is basically a headband that monitors eye movements and starts blinking low levels of light, which become incorporated into our dream when we enter the REM sleep stage associated with dreaming, without waking one up.

LaBerge's work is summarized in his popular book *Lucid Dreaming,* which I highly recommend. In 1987 LaBerge founded the Lucidity Institute, an organization that promotes research into lucid dreaming as well as running courses for the general public on how to achieve a lucid dream. In lucid dreams one has the power to make almost anything happen. One can even change the dream environment by closing the eyes in the dream and spinning around in circles, imagining where he or she would like to be. When the subject opens his or her eyes, I've found, there he or she is. When I interviewed LaBerge, I asked him about the relationship between a computer-simulated virtual reality and lucid dreaming. He said that lucid dreaming was like "high-resolution virtual reality."

Several Hollywood films have explored this idea, such as *Inception, Waking Life, and Vanilla Sky.* How other species and advanced extraterrestrials might experience lucid dreaming fascinates me. The dream life of dolphins in particular is a subject that has long intrigued me, because they have such sophisticated brains and sleep in a manner very different from us; only half of their brain sleeps at a time. I've wondered if they experience lucid dreams as a significant part of their reality and what it's like for them as well as for big-brained whales and elephants.

Researchers from the Max Planck Institutes of Psychiatry in Munich have shown which centers of the brain become active when we become aware of ourselves in dreams, exhibiting what the researchers call "meta-consciousness."

Studies employing magnetic resonance tomography (MRT) compared the activity of the brain during lucid dreaming with the activity measured immediately before in a normal dream. This allowed the researchers to identify the characteristic brain activities of lucid awareness.

The researchers demonstrated that a specific network in the brain—the right dorsolateral prefrontal cortex, the frontopolar regions, and the precuneus—is activated when lucidity is attained. All of these brain regions are associated with self-reflective functions, and this new insight may help us to understand the neural basis of human consciousness.

PERSONAL EXPERIENCES WITH LUCID DREAMING

I've personally had an enormous amount of experience with lucid dreaming, more than anyone else I've ever met. Thanks to the use of several psychoactive compounds, I've had many dozens of prolonged lucid dreams, some of which have lasted for hours or even whole nights at a time. Although I've had spontaneous lucid dreams since I was a child, they began to increase in frequency after I started using psychedelics and practicing techniques that I learned from LaBerge.

The best techniques that I learned for increasing my frequency of lucid dreams is to increase my dream recall by always writing down my dreams upon waking and by getting into the regular habit of asking myself, "Am I dreaming right now? How do I know?" If one gets into the habit of questioning this while one is in a waking state, I've found that the habit carries over into one's dream life. However, usually something bizarre in the dream will trigger the thought, *Is this a dream?* Then, if I suspect that I'm dreaming, I test my environment to make sure.

The three best tests that I know of for determining if I'm in a lucid dream, which have been confirmed by others, are as follows:

1. Look at some written material in a book or on a piece of paper. Then look away and look back. If you're dreaming the text will have changed, every time.
2. Turn off a light switch. In a dream, the light in the room will remain on after the switch has been turned off.
3. Try to fly. This may take some effort at first, but if I'm dreaming I can always manage to become airborne with several leaps into the air.

Once I've confirmed that I'm dreaming I'm simply delighted beyond words and have explored these alternative worlds in great detail over the years. One of the very first things that I did in lucid dreams was to examine my hands. It seems that establishing good hand-eye coordination when entering new states of consciousness is instinctive and adaptive. There are more nerves connecting your eyes and your hands than any other two parts of the human body.

While writing my science-fiction novel *Virus: The Alien Strain,* I tried to think of an alternative phrase for the commonly used idiom *I know it like the back of my hand,* and I realized that there was nothing that I've seen more often throughout my entire life than the back of my own hand. (I ended up going with *as familiar as the sound of my own breath.*) I've noticed that babies often appear to study their hands, as do lucid dreamers, psychedelic trippers, and people in virtual reality when entering these states of consciousness or simulated environments for the first time.

Besides noticing that LSD and MDMA can sometimes trigger lucid dreams several days after the experience I've also learned that a number of other drugs can increase the likelihood of having lucid dreams, some quite reliably and for hours at a time, like consecutively repeated sleep doses of GBL, an analog of GHB, and strong doses of opiates or poppy tea. Some herbs that enhance dreaming, such as *Calea zacatechichi,* can also be helpful, as can periods of sleep deprivation. The ketamine experiences that I had, which I described earlier, were a lot like lucid dreams. Isolation tanks can also be effective tools for enhancing lucidity in one's dreams.

When I asked LaBerge what kind of techniques he thought were the most effective for producing lucid dreams, he replied:

> If you were to say, "I want to become a lucid dreamer, how should I go about it?" I would say that means you've got some extra time and energy in your life, some unallocated attention that you could apply to working on this. If you're somebody that's so busy that you have hardly time to take a walk, you're not going to have the time and energy to do this. We have developed a course in lucid dreaming that is designed for people to use at home. The first lesson in there is about how you develop dream recall. After you've got a sufficient level of dream recall you start studying your dreams for the dream signs; what's dreamlike about them? You then start doing exercises that use your focus in your mind on your typical dream content, becoming more reflective and developing your ability to have specific

intentions that you carry out in the future and so on. The course in lucid dreaming right now is something you can use either with or without a DreamLight, which is a device we developed primarily in response to people's requests for methods to help them have lucid dreams. It's a mask that you wear while you're asleep and it flashes a light during REM, not so much as to wake you up but enough to remind you in your dream that you are dreaming.

When I first discovered how to embark on lucid dreams at will, with pretty good consistency, I began to experiment with what was possible, with all the expected enthusiasm of a child set free in a candy shop. All my first adventures, unsurprisingly, involved an unbridled indulgence in wild sexual escapades with pretty girls and flying through exotic landscapes, usually close to the ground, which I find especially fun. Flying doesn't come easy to me in lucid dreams; it takes considerable effort. I have to concentrate really hard and very slowly elevate myself off the ground, and then as I maintain this state, I rise faster and fly farther but must continue to concentrate on what I'm doing or I start to fall. I indulged in lots of wild and forbidden sex in lucid dreams, with multiple partners, and flying to my heart's content, before I started to wonder about other possibilities.

Next I tried doing psychedelic drugs in dreams—cannabis, LSD, ketamine, salvia, and DMT—all with effects that were consistent with those I've experienced while awake, albeit somewhat milder and somewhat weirder, because I'm already in a different state of consciousness when I'm dreaming and my natural DMT levels are likely elevated. These experiences suggest that the drugs may not really be necessary to have the experiences they're so often used to create as one's brain seems to be able to re-create the experiences in a dream—unless, perhaps, one is actually doing "astral drugs" in the dreams, real drugs that are composed of some exotic type of dark matter in a parallel universe, which is having a psychopharmacological effect on our multidimensional "dream brains."

One of the next things that I tried exploring in a lucid dream was what happens to consciousness after death. I reasoned that if I could (safely) commit suicide in a dream, then I may gain some insight into what actually happens to consciousness after death. So, after thinking about this possibility, the next time I found myself in a lucid dream, I remembered what I wanted to do. After confirming repeatedly that I was indeed dreaming—more so than usual—I conveniently found a handgun located in my right hand. I took the gun, pointed at the side of my head, and bravely pulled the trigger. After the bullet fired, the next thing I knew I was bodiless, in a dark silent void, alone with just my thoughts. It wasn't unpleasant, but it was certainly much less dramatic than what I was expecting.

In another series of lucid dreams one night I found myself repeatedly floating up toward the ceiling of a strange room, out of my body—only it wasn't happening in material reality; it was happening in a lucid dream. I was having an out-of-the-dream-body experience.

In later lucid dreams I began to make friends and seemingly establish relationships with the other people I met there. When I tried to describe to these people that we were in a lucid dream, at first they were almost all very resistant to this idea. They most certainly didn't think that they were merely aspects of me! When I showed some people in a dream that I could fly, they got upset and tried to pull me back down to the ground. However, later I was able to teach others how to fly too. I find it interesting that all of my dreams always seem to involve other people. I can't remember a single dream I ever had where I was completely alone—except my suicide lucid dream—even though in my waking life, making my living as a writer, I spend much of my time alone.

As my lucid dreams became more and more frequent, I met people who made me question the reality of my lucid dreams and whether they were all fabricated by my own brain—similar to my experiences with DMT. It seems as though this place in my brain where lucid dreaming is occurring is an independently existing alternative reality where some people live their day-to-day lives and others whom I've met there seem to be like me—other dreamers who temporarily come to this place through the process of lucid dreaming. I once met someone in a lucid dream who also recognized that we were in a dream, and we excitedly grasped one another's shoulders and looked into one another's eyes, exclaiming, "Wow! We're in a dream! This is so cool!" We were in total disbelief that we could be there together, inside a place that we got to through dreaming! It seemed totally impossible, but, nonetheless, there we were.

I've had lucid dreams where I seemingly spend hours carefully observing the details of small objects, trying hard to tell if there's any way to determine if this dream reality is any less real than the reality that I construct in consensus material reality here on planet Earth. However, the laws of physics in these dream states, which also seem consistent, appear to vary from the laws here, which makes this difficult to determine. My mind has a much more powerful influence there, more directly and immediately than in my waking material reality state. I can rub my hands over people's faces in lucid dreams and change what they look like. Everything is much more mutable there. I've tried staring at written words in lucid dreams, deliberately trying to get them to stay consistent, to no avail; they always change in a few seconds before my eyes.

I've tried on numerous attempts to form some type of alliance with fellow dreamers that I've met in lucid dreams, by trying to exchange our earthly names and contact information. So far, I've found this to be completely impossible, almost as though a law of physics in this other reality was preventing me from doing so. For some reason I find it impossible to tell other lucid dreamers that my name is David Jay Brown or that I live in California, even though I can clearly think this in my mind at the time.

Every time I've tried, the words simply would not come out, and everyone else in the dream appears to have the same difficulty. In one lucid dream, when I was trying to exchange contact information with a fellow dream character, he suddenly got the bright idea to write it down on a piece of paper. *Brilliant!* I thought. Why hadn't I thought of that? However, when he handed me the piece of paper and I looked at it, the letters were, of course, continuously changing and almost seemed to be mocking my attempt to understand them.

For example, I would look at the paper and see a long string of strange and obscure, ever-shifting symbols, some in English and some in what looked like alien hieroglyphics. But then at the end of the letters would be a comma followed by *M.D.* It was like some higher order of intelligence was preventing this type of exchange and even making fun of my attempt to do so. I have literally tried for hours (confirmed by my physical reality clock) in lucid dreams to exchange contact information with others to no avail, but I haven't given up yet!

It may be that after we die, we move into a dream world of our own creation during this life, and in that world we would be "God." It may be that we're all evolving into gods.

HOW IT FEELS TO BECOME A DEITY

When I consider the fractal, holographic nature of the universe, an interesting perspective arises with regard to my lucid dreams when I contemplate the archetypal role of the messiah in Western religions. The messiah is generally thought of as God incarnating him/herself as a human being—one imbued with seemingly infinite wisdom and power. So, then, the messiah—whose total self is holographically represented as a smaller self within the context of all the mini selves that make up the specialized components of one's brain and body—would appear as you, the lucid dreamer in your dream reality. A messiah in our consensual shared material reality could probably manifest in the same way when "God" has a lucid dream. Of course, psychedelics and mystical states of consciousness teach us that we're all ultimately one universal being, so there's a paradox and a joke in here somewhere that's hard for us to fully grasp with our three-dimensional monkey brains.

Nonetheless, this is how I feel in my lucid dreams, like I'm the messiah in the world of my inner selves. Because all of life itself may be something like a dream of sorts, as Hindu philosophy suggests, it makes sense that a representation of the whole of which we are all a part could manifest among us and seem to have the same incredible power and knowledge that this is all just a dream, a manifestation of our minds that one can easily change at will.

What humans think of as God may just be the "person" that we all live inside of, a cosmic version of ourselves, and, perhaps, like us all, someone afflicted with a bit of multiple-personality disorder. Our whole universe may be his or her mind, and when he/she becomes lucid in his/her dreams—that is, our reality—then he or she would manifest in our world as a being of unlimited power and wisdom. Jesus, Mohammed, Zeus, Superman, and Neo in *The Matrix* come to mind as some of the archetypal manifestations of this intuition.

I learned in one lucid dream that I was able to move small objects with the power of my mind simply by looking at them and willing them to move. I could make the objects zip across the floor; I just had to focus on one and I could deliberately make it glide across the floor by imagining and willing it to do so. In another lucid dream someone looked at me intently and I suddenly fell over on the floor. He was laughing at me, and I knew that he had done it to me somehow. Remembering that I could move things with my mind in a previous lucid dream, I looked intently at him and then made him fall over backward onto a couch full of pillows! I felt like a superhero with a new superpower and began knocking over other people in the dream just to prank them.

I've experienced long, prolonged periods of lucid dreaming where I repeatedly return to the same place with the same people. The vividness and clarity of this place is every bit as convincing and stable as this reality, with some minor exceptions. With some effort I can float, fly, or move objects with my mind, and people can transform into other people. I can carefully examine and feel objects with great detail and precision. Technologies there always appear slightly different from how they do in our reality. For example, the keys on keyboard displays are different and the symbols change oddly, like they're alive. These lucid dreams seem to me like what have been described as parallel universes.

I can sometimes stay in these lucid dream states for up to six hours at a time, waking up and falling asleep over and over, without ever losing consciousness. Maintaining a state of lucid awareness during the process of going from waking to sleeping—without losing any continuity of consciousness—can be an extremely pleasurable experience, more blissful and ecstatic than any drug I've ever done. I've had such fun and beautiful experiences in lucid dreams that sometimes I didn't want them to end. One morning I really didn't want to return to this world and, knowing that I didn't have much time left there and that the lucid dream would end soon, I frantically ran around in the dream world asking everyone I encountered if they knew how I could stay there, without waking up in this reality.

No one seemed to know. Finally I encountered this beautiful, wise black woman wearing a colorful flowing dress. She simply smiled at me and pointed to her stomach, which revealed that she was pregnant. I immediately understood what she meant, that the only way to stay there was to be born there as a baby and that this place attracts souls from all over the multiverse. Then she dissolved, and I woke up clutching my pillow. Months later I had another lucid dream where I encountered the same wise and beautiful black woman in the back of a car we were riding in together, and again I pleaded with her to tell me how I could stay there. She smiled at me and lovingly said, "I'll see you when you get home."

Over time my experiences with lucid dreaming have become much more stable and prolonged without any chemical assistance, and I'm just left with my jaw hanging open for an explanation. I sometimes feel like I'm living lives in several dimensions simultaneously, like the late spirit medium Jane Roberts wrote about in her novel *The Education of Oversoul Seven* and psychonaut Zoe7 writes about in his *Into the Void* trilogy.

Another thing that I've learned to enjoy doing in lucid dreams is going to sleep in the lucid dream and then having a lucid dream within the lucid dream. This can be done repeatedly so that one is consciously dreaming within dreams within dreams, and I find that the laws of physics get progressively more and more bizarre in each successive layer of the lucid dream. I wonder if this is what the Tibetan Buddhists refer to as the different levels of dream yoga. My only concern in doing this is that I may get so deep into these other realities that I'll get lost and won't be able to find my way back to this one!

I wonder if these dream states are really independently existing realities or merely the constructs of my own mind. They seem every bit as convincing to my lucid, rational, conscious mind, which completely remembers this reality while I'm there, and advanced physics leaves plenty of latitude for the possibility that these experiences have a genuine basis in reality. That is, assuming that this reality is truly real.

I suspect that true communication with other beings in dream states may be genuinely possible. I've had what appeared to be shared dreams and seemingly telepathically shared, psychedelic visions with people whom I'm close with, and there have been some uncanny similarities. Stephan LaBerge's lucid-dream research and Stanley Krippner's telepathy-dream research may just be hinting at the kind of incredible dream research that our future holds in store for us.

SHARED DREAMING EXPERIENCES

I've shared dreams with people over the years with whom I've been closely bonded—or so it seemed—although so far none of these have been lucid. When we were children, for example, my brother and I once dreamed that we were aboard a spaceship together, where we encountered our grandmother with birthday cake in her hair. I asked LaBerge about the possibility of shared dreams. He replied:

> I haven't really experimented with that. I consider it to be theoretically possible, but it's not something that I felt was of developmental value first of all. There are many aspects of dream control that I haven't pursued. I've emphasized controlling myself and my responses to what happens instead of making it magically different, because I've wanted something that would generalize the waking state. In this world we don't have the power to magically make other people appear and disappear. There have been a few people who've said, "I can visit you in your dream," and I've said, "Okay do so." But I've never experienced an unequivocal success that I remember. I think the problem is that we tend to bring mental models from the waking state into the dream state. So we have expectations in the dream, especially in a lucid dream. Here it is, it's all so real, and so hey! you two people look perfectly real to me so you'll remember this conversation later, right? Now why would I think you'd do that, any more than I would think this table would remember this conversation? One of the things you have to do in developing skill with lucid dreaming is to be critical of your state of mind. So you wake up from a lucid dream and you think, did I make some assumptions that were inappropriate or do something that didn't make sense? So you can therefore refine and clarify your thinking and build up mental models that are appropriate to the dream world. I dreamt in a lucid dream that I was flying above the San Francisco Bay, and I had the thought, my body is asleep over there, I'll go visit it. And I woke and said, what? This is a dream! Your body's not in there or you'd be in trouble if your body's asleep in your own dream, how could you wake up? People who don't make that extra effort don't tend to learn.

Nonetheless, my experience with shared dreaming, and reports from others, lead me to also suspect that they may really be possible. In the future I think that a sophisticated science of exploring alternative realities through lucid dreaming will be developed.

Some psychedelics, particularly ketamine, DMT, and *Salvia divinorum,* can reliably produce out-of-body, lucid-dream-like experiences. I asked John Lilly about this once. Ever the trickster, here is our dialogue on the subject:

DAVID: Do you see a similarity between lucid dreaming and ketamine experiences?

JOHN: No. Lucid dreaming is never as powerful as ketamine.

DAVID: Well, one nice thing about ketamine is that you can maintain the high for as long as you want.

JOHN: When people start talking about higher states of consciousness I say, "In outer space there's no up or down."

DAVID: It all becomes relative.

JOHN: No, it isn't even relative.

DAVID: It isn't even relative?

JOHN: It isn't anything you can describe.

DAVID: Now I'm thoroughly confused.

JOHN: If you stay around me long enough you're going to get a whole new language.

A lot of people have lucid dreams after they learn about them—so don't be surprised if you have one tonight! And to respond to LaBerge's statement that "this table would remember this conversation" I would call upon my experiences with the psychedelic plant *Salvia divinorum,* which seemed to imply that everything, including what we usually think of as inanimate objects, are actually alive and conscious. We'll be discussing this in chapter 5.

Meanwhile, just discovering that all of the parts of my own brain and body I had previously thought were unconscious were actually conscious, and independently minded to some degree, was mind-boggling enough for me to cope with. It seems that our brains contain a number of different types of intelligence.

5
Models of the Mind and Interpreting Psychedelic Experiences

Neuroscientists Roger Sperry and Michael Gazzaniga have demonstrated that not only are the right and left hemispheres of the brain relatively independently functioning but that many submodules in our brain act like mini brains, with their own agendas. What's most surprising is that although we can scientifically demonstrate that brain modules operate relatively independently and influence our actions in ways our conscious mind remains unaware, we tend to rationalize why we make the choices that we do, citing reasons that often have nothing to do with the real cause.

Let me give you an example. In people who suffer from severe temporal lobe epilepsy, in some cases the bundle of nerve fibers that connect the right and left hemispheres, known as the corpus callosum, is surgically severed so that an epileptic seizure won't spread from one hemisphere to the other. The surgeries have been relatively successful, but there have been some very strange consequences. I've seen videos of people who have had the split-brain operation, and it seems like two people are now residing in their brain. Sometimes one part of the body is trying to put on a pair of pants while the other side is trying to take them off.

One particularly striking example of how split-brain patients see the world was made clear in an experiment by Roger Sperry. As most people know, the right side of the body is controlled by the left hemisphere of the brain, and the left side of the body is controlled by the right side of the brain. Within the human eye our visual field is split as well, with the left half of the image going to the right side of the brain and the right half of the image going to the left side of the brain.

Sperry designed an apparatus that allowed him to project an image to one half of the eye at a time so that the visual information signals just went to one side of the brain. When the subject saw the image with his right visual field, this went to the left hemisphere of his brain, where the language center is. When asked what he saw, the subject could easily say what it was. However, when the image was projected on to his left visual field and traveled to the right hemisphere of the brain, the subject would say that they had no memory of seeing anything.

Surprisingly, when the subject was asked to pick out the object that he saw from a pile of different objects, with his left hand, which is controlled by the right side of the brain, he could easily do so. The strangest finding of all came when the subjects were asked why they had chosen that object from the pile when they said they didn't see anything. All of the subjects came up with reasons that had nothing to do with the reality of having perceived it with their right hemisphere. "It reminded me of a toy from my childhood" or "It just seemed interesting" were typical responses.

Learning about this work in graduate school led me to the conclusion that the unified feeling of self that I generally equate with myself is largely incomplete and mostly illusory. Psychedelics have certainly taught me how mutable my mind is when I shift the neurochemistry in my brain. I've learned that within my mind are many minds, and that my ego-mind is nestled within a larger, far more encompassing species-mind, and that all minds are forever nestled like fractals within ever-larger minds. With this understanding comes the realization that there are many different levels to intelligence.

INTELLIGENCE, THE EIGHT-CIRCUIT
MODEL OF THE BRAIN,
AND NEURAL IMPRINTING

How do we define *intelligence*? I think Timothy Leary's model of intelligence is among the best. He uses the neuron—an individual brain cell—as a model for understanding intelligence, which can be divided into three functional stages: reception, integration, and transmission. Thus intelligence can be defined as the most efficient way to receive, process, and communicate information.

Every brain cell is composed of three anatomical parts: a cell body with the nucleus, a large axon that receives information from other neurons, and smaller branching dendrites that communicate information to other neurons via electrochemical signals. Leary applied this model to intelligence, which can thus be increased in three ways: by expanding the scope of the information one receives, by more efficiently and creatively processing and remembering this information, and then more effectively communicating what you have learned to others. These three stages create a continual feedback loop whereby intelligence is progressively increased and expanded.

I think one of Leary's most important contributions to psychology was his theoretical model of the eight-circuit brain, and this is one of the best models for understanding what happens to us during a psychedelic experience. This model has helped me understand my psychedelic experiences better than any of the traditional psychological models from Freud and Jung to Maslow and Grof. Leary postulates eight basic types of intelligence.

I mentioned earlier that Leary attempted to show that life on Earth evolves in the same way that many other dynamic processes in the universe develop, according to the law of octaves and the periodic table of elements, and that we can surmise that this pattern is likely to occur all over the universe, wherever life evolves. This idea was the basis for Leary's development of the eight-circuit model of the brain. The law of octaves shows that what we perceive as the rainbow, the visible color spectrum, or the range of musical notes, is the key to understanding how many processes in the universe progress—from the life cycles of stars to the colors that a wound goes through when it heals, as well as to human development and evolution. This idea deserves further exploration, and it was Leary's stroke of brilliance to apply the law of octaves to the evolution of consciousness.

Drawing from both mystical and scientific systems, Leary tried to show in numerous books that the human brain/mind is basically composed of eight fundamental circuits—individual minds or neural modules—that correspond to the law of octaves. The first four brain circuits, or stages of human development, are focused on survival and establishing a firm foundation in physical reality. Whatever the environmental circumstances are when these circuits first emerge will imprint the circuit with a basic positive or negative association that has long-lasting psychological consequences. What follows is a brief summary of the eight-circuit model of the brain, which has been further developed by Robert Anton Wilson, Antero Alli, and Karl Jansen.

Circuit 1

Circuit 1 is the biosurvival circuit, which is common to all living organisms. I suspect that in animals this anatomically corresponds to the brainstem, the oldest and most primitive part of the brain, which is primarily focused on breathing, eating, sleeping, and monitoring physiological functions. Circuit 1 responds to environmental stimuli with fight or flight, with individual survival always being the primary concern.

This was the first nervous-system circuit to evolve, and it always takes the highest priority because it was obviously "chosen" by natural selection. "Live or die!" is this circuit's motto, and genes that encoded for an ambivalence about bodily survival perished long ago. This circuit is activated at birth, and many people have imprinted this state with a sense of danger, when the optimal state would be one of safety. This imprint determines our primary orientation toward life, whether we see life as largely good or bad, and much of our personality values derive from this orientation. Medicine emerged from the first circuit.

Circuit 2

Circuit 2 is the emotional and empathy circuit. I suspect that this corresponds to the limbic system in the brain and the amygdala, which are primarily concerned with emotional responses, pecking orders, and social bonding. This circuit emerged on Earth when the first vertebrates evolved into mammals. Embarrassment, attachment, love, caring, anger, sadness, happiness, confidence, and other emotions are developed when this circuit is activated as a toddler—when one starts to see oneself in the context of others who need to be negotiated with. We begin to realize that other people have feelings like we do. Among other social practices, this is where politics derives from. Many people have imprinted this state with fear and insecurity when the optimal state is love and confidence.

Circuit 3

Circuit 3 is the cognitive circuit. I suspect that this corresponds primarily to the left hemisphere of the brain, which is largely concerned with language, mathematics, symbolic communication, and linear thought. This circuit emerged on our planet with the first tool-using primates, and it is activated in individual development when we learn how to speak. It is later refined when we learn to read, write, and perform mathematical calculations. This circuit is what most people mean by the term *intelligence,* and it's these neural functions that are generally tested in so-called IQ tests. A positive imprint with this circuit gives people the impression that they're generally smart. Science and technology emerged from this circuit.

Circuit 4

Circuit 4 is the social/sexual circuit. I suspect that this corresponds to the left frontal cortex of the brain, and it is largely concerned with our gender and role in organized societies. This circuit emerged on our planet when the first social organisms evolved and individuals became free to specialize and develop their unique abilities. In human beings it's activated at puberty, when we begin to see ourselves as vital components of the larger social structures that support our existence, and in this stage of our development we find specialized functions that we largely identify with as ourselves. Ask the average adult human being at a party what they do, and you'll generally get a fourth-circuit response. This is also the circuit that allows us to form romantic and sexual partnerships with one another, and it encourages a strong allegiance to the human hive, which can be seen among elderly church and temple attendees.

According to Leary and Wilson, these are the larval or terrestrial circuits of the brain that appear developmentally in sequence as we grow—recapitulating our stages of evolution—and specific drugs also activate them. For example, opiates activate circuit 1; strong doses of alcohol activate circuit 2; caffeine, cocaine, amphetamines, hydergine and other cognitive enhancers activate circuit 3; and low doses of alcohol, phenibut, MDMA, and Valium activate circuit 4. The situations that we were in when these circuits were first activated imprint us with that orientation.

The second four circuits, or states of consciousness, recapitulate the information processed in the first four circuits at a level that transcends mere physical survival and that opens the door to creativity, pleasure, fun, philosophy, psychic phenomena, out-of-body experiences, and spirituality. They represent our possibilities for future evolution, the fruits of our survival.

Circuit 5

Circuit 5 is the neurosomatic circuit. I suspect that this generally refers to the right hemisphere of the brain, especially the right frontal lobe, which is concerned with whole-pattern recognition, intuition, and creativity. This circuit emerged on our planet when groups of social organisms solved the problems of survival and terrestrial navigation, such as in dolphins, whales, bonobos, and some privileged human beings.

When fully activated this brain circuit is experienced as exquisitely heightened sensory sensitivity that brings bliss and rapture with the slightest pleasure. However, this circuit can also amplify painful feelings, so one needs to learn how to use it skillfully. This aesthetically sensitive circuit is activated by cannabis, MDMA, meditation, massage, certain types of music, hot tubs, yoga, and tantra. Mind/body medicine, art, music, and dance emerged from this circuit.

Circuit 6

Circuit 6 is the neuroelectric circuit, or metaprogramming awareness, as John Lilly called it. I suspect that this circuit is located in an area of the brain known as the reticular activating system, which acts as a kind of filtering system in the brain. As with the following two circuits, this circuit emerged on our planet when shamans in indigenous societies began using psychedelic plants, and it allows us to consciously make new imprints on all of the circuits that developed earlier by relaxing the inhibitions of our neural censoring mechanisms. When activated it reveals all of reality to be a simulation created by our own brains, similar to Neo's awakening about the nature of what he had thought to be reality in the film *The Matrix,* only open to our conscious reconfiguration.

People often describe this state of consciousness as ego death. This is where our usual personalities dissolve and a boundless state of consciousness replaces it. Telepathy, synchronicity, and instructive or meaningful closed-eye visions are commonly reported in this state of consciousness. LSD, psilocybin, mescaline, isolation tanks, and computer-simulated realities are specific triggers for opening this system so that much of the information that is normally censored from the higher cortex— especially the prefrontal cortex—of the brain is allowed to freely flow. This gives us the opportunity to rewire our conditioned thinking and make new neural imprints. In this circuit we realize that we are ultimately responsible for creating our own realities. Developments in neural plasticity, personal computers, the Internet, and virtual reality emerged from this circuit.

Circuit 7

Circuit 7 is the neurogenetic circuit, or phylogenetic consciousness, as Stanislav Groff calls it. I discussed this circuit in detail in the first chapter of this book, because it has been a primary guiding force in my life. I think that the center for this awareness lies deeper than the brain, inside the nucleus of brain cells, within the DNA molecule itself, which resonates with the entire web of life on this planet and elsewhere. Ayahuasca and high doses of LSD or psilocybin activate this circuit, which allows us to communicate with the genetic intelligence that sustains the global biosphere and see the world from a mythic or archetypal perspective.

Powerful dreams with universal themes may sometimes be important clues from this collective unconscious, as Jung called circuit 7. People commonly describe this state of consciousness in spiritual or mystical terms, and it is often a vital component in what people generally describe as a religious experience, although that also usually involves the activation of circuit eight.

Some of the very best literary descriptions of this state of consciousness can be found in the book *The Cosmic Serpent,* by anthropologist Jeremy Narby, which seeks to explain the relationship between the twisting, coiling snakes often seen in ayahuasca visions and the biochemistry of the DNA molecule. The Human Genome Project, genetic engineering, myths, and archetypal fairy tales emerged from this circuit. And isn't it interesting that the two most important discoveries made in genetics in the past century—the structure of the DNA molecule by Francis Crick, and the development of PCR by Kary Mullis—were reportedly catalyzed by the use of LSD?

Francis Crick also developed a lesser-known theory to help explain the origin of life on Earth called directed panspermia, which is summarized in his book *Life Itself,* and also seems to be inspired by the seventh circuit. Crick hypothesizes that extraterrestrial spores traveling through space on the back of meteorites seed planets throughout the galaxies, similar to Terence McKenna's idea about psilocybin mushroom spores traveling among the stars.

Circuit 8

Circuit 8 is the neuroatomic or quantum nonlocal circuit. I suspect that the locus for this state of consciousness is in the center of the atom, or perhaps within smaller, more centralized—and, paradoxically, more nonlocalized—subatomic particles. This is the circuit where out-of-body experiences and interdimensional journeys are experienced, or where one achieves a state of supreme union with the whole universe. A circuit 7 religious experience is felt as a sense of unity with all life, whereas a circuit 8 religious experience is often reported as a sense of unity with the entire cosmos, all that exists.

As with the two previous circuits, this circuit came under our conscious control when shamans in indigenous societies began using psychedelic plants, although it is also naturally activated during near-death experiences. Specific pharmacological triggers for this circuit include high doses of DMT, salvia, ketamine, and MXE. Nanotechnology (atomic engineering) and the Singularity emerged from this circuit.

The universal developmental sequence expressed in this model of consciousness and intelligence helps us to understand where we might be going as we enter the Singularity, as each of the different brain circuits corresponds to specific scientific, medical, technological, and philosophical breakthroughs for our species. One can only guess where future-evolving circuits 9 through 16 might take us, but, presumably, they will follow the same developmental pattern that we see with the law of octaves.

Within the framework of this system Leary also suggested that human beings might be born into different social castes, like social insects are, and that our basic personality types may be akin to what in social insects corresponds to workers, drones, queens, and so forth. If this is true then it seems like the science and art of astrology may be a primitive attempt to classify the basic human personality castes. I think that there may be something to astrology.

Astronomers are quick to point out that the gravity from earthbound objects has a greater influence on us than the stars and planets do. However, I don't think it's the effects from these celestial objects in the heavens that are creating the different personality types; rather, it appears that some people have noticed that there is a correlation between the configuration of celestial objects in the sky and the birth of certain types of people. In other words: as above, so below. Whatever the cosmic forces that influence the configuration of the stars might be, they could also be influencing our personality patterns. For example, it may be that seasonal variations in solar activity affect our DNA at conception, and then this determines which type of personality pattern is chosen for a particular nervous system.

Understanding how different brain circuits function in our nervous system gives us insight into the matrix of multiple selves that make up who we are. (Circuits run energy and information round and round in circles, I realized on a shamanic journey, which helps to explain much of human behavior.) MIT computer scientist Marvin Minsky's book *Society of Mind* and neuroscientist Michael Gazzaniga's book *The Social Brain* both describe how individual modules in the brain can operate largely independently from one another without our conscious awareness. We all have multiple personalities. However, for some people these personalities aren't well integrated.

MY EXPERIENCE WITH MULTIPLE PERSONALITY ORDER AND DISORDER

When I was in my midtwenties working as a psychiatric counselor I had the opportunity to develop close relationships with two remarkable women who suffered from multiple personality disorder (MPD). Both of these women had suffered from horrifically traumatic episodes that occurred when they were very young, too young to have formed a coherently organized sense of self. My experiences with these women became the inspiration for my science-fiction novel *Virus: The*

Alien Strain, which was written through the eyes of someone who suffers from MPD.

MPD is a sometimes debilitating, dissociative psychiatric disorder that is caused by severe physical and/or emotional trauma at an age so young that a unified personality never emerges from the brain as it develops. Instead, numerous—simply a few to many hundreds—of relatively independently existing personalities form to compete for control of the brain. Each personality is almost like a unique person, with a specific function, and consistent perspective and individual sense of self, complete with personal memories, and even unique medical conditions, reactions to drugs, allergies, eye color, and independent dreams at night. It really is an uncanny and truly mysterious phenomenon.

A strange and powerful synchronicity highlights my relationship with one of these women, increasing the uncanniness of all this. Let's call the first woman I met Rebekkah, which was the name of one of her alters (alternative personalities), of which she had hundreds. There were even personalities within her that suffered from MPD, that is, personalities within personalities within personalities, like opening a Russian nesting doll or zooming in on a mathematical fractal.

During the late 1980s while I was writing *Brainchild,* I was working for a suicide hotline in Santa Cruz where I would counsel psychologically desperate people with intense emotional problems, and who were in crisis and just barely hanging on to their lives. Rebekkah called repeatedly, and we spoke for hours as she switched between alternate personalities—some of whom were suicidal and threatened all of the other alters' survival. Surprisingly, the alters didn't even realize that they were all personalities occupying the same body! Some of the alters actually thought that other alters were other people living in separate bodies.

Rebekkah was an exceptionally bright woman with a dissociative disorder that utterly fascinated me, so we spoke for long periods of time, beyond what was necessary for the service that I was doing. I was simply astonished by how unique each personality seemed. Rebekkah was living somewhere in the Midwest when I first met her. In 1988, after we spoke a number of times, I made arrangements for her to be admitted to a psychiatric hospital in Los Angeles, where she began her treatment. After she was admitted to the hospital I didn't have any contact with her for several years.

In 1989 I moved to Topanga Canyon, a small mountain town outside of Los Angeles, and I started a doctoral program in behavioral neuroscience at USC. Shortly after leaving this program in the early 1990s I began working as a counselor with a psychiatric treatment agency that treated recovering schizophrenic, dissociative, and borderline patients in a residential setting. On my first day at the new treatment center I was introduced to the patient whom I would be counseling. When I heard her name and diagnosis, my jaw simply dropped. By pure coincidence or synchronicity, Rebekkah and I would be working together for the following year.

The time when I was working with Rebekkah coincided with the year I spent regularly doing ketamine with John Lilly on the weekends, and I couldn't help but think that the dissociative effects of the drug were giving me insight into Rebekkah's condition. These ideas were fictionalized in my novel *Virus: The Alien Strain,* as I learned just how flexible and mutable the gestalts of one's personalities truly are.

Rebekkah was an amazing human being. She had hundreds of different, independently functioning alters, each with their own unique way of seeing the world. Each alter was permanently frozen at a specific age and at a particular stage of development. Astonishingly, they each had their own medical allergies (that would miraculously vanish when she switched personalities) and even personal, individual dreams at night. Sometimes her eye color would change when she switched personalities. It truly seemed like a paranormal occurrence whenever she would switch, because I really felt like I was with different people. She would have to have been an extremely dedicated and unusually talented Academy Award–winning actress to pull this off if it wasn't real.

Rebekkah claimed to have been raised in a satanic cult and relayed an enormous amount of details to support her eyebrow-raising claim, which truly brought these experiences into the Twilight Zone. I never knew what to make of this or of the horrific stories she told about her childhood, but clearly something deeply traumatic happened to her. Our psychiatric team was forced to monitor her phone calls, because it appeared that some people who called her could make her do things against her will, like suicide attempts, just by saying certain coded words.

When I later saw reports of other people with MPD diagnoses making very similar claims I really had to wonder if these cults could be real. While I'm not sure what to make of all this, the skeptics' immediate dismissal of these claims overlooks some really powerful, strangely compelling, and extremely disturbing evidence. It may be archetypal, or something other than literal, but something truly weird is going on when people with MPD make claims that they've been raised in satanic cults. Without personal experience I never would have suspected this to be the case. Who knows what human beings are capable of? We certainly know that they're prone to bizarre beliefs and that they sometimes act in fanatical ways.

Another woman whom I'll call Layla also repeatedly called the suicide hotline I worked at. I broke the rules with Layla, and we became close personal friends—something forbidden in the therapeutic world of psychology. But I was so fascinated by her mind, her creativity, her intelligence, and her strange psychological disorder that I spent time hanging out with her. One of her alters' names was Layla, and she was a beautiful woman in her early twenties when I met her.

I spent innumerable hours on the phone with Layla and visited with her a number of times. She was an extremely intelligent and unusually creative woman who had a young, suicidal, and promiscuous alter that got her into all kinds of trouble. I would watch in astonishment when I was with her as she would simultaneously compose a beautiful letter with one hand while her other hand uncannily drew a perfect portrait. She had an extraordinary ability to divide the functions of her brain like no else I had ever seen.

The best book that I've seen on the subject of MPD is called *When*

Rabbit Howls, which was written by someone with MPD, so all of the different selves helped to coauthor the book. The author is listed as a community: The Troops for Truddi Chase.

It genuinely seems like each alter in someone who suffers from MPD is a unique person. It really is uncanny and undeniable, but how can this possibly be? Is the MPD patient possessed by more spirits than the rest of us, or is something else happening? This really helps us get at the core question of who we really are. The cause of this disorder is always the same: severe and repeated physical or emotional trauma prior to age one. I think this prevents a consistent, integrated field of consciousness from organizing our brain's activity into a whole pattern, so myriad competing states form with only relative stability, each with cooperating functions. Personalities are formed, for example, to be able to function in certain social situations and are called forth by some overseeing, organizing personality when needed, or by overwhelming stress.

I think the brain/mind system is a microcosm of everything that exists and that reflecting on the nature of MPD can lead us to great insight about how our individual minds are like reflections of the whole universe. I've had experiences with LSD where it seemed like my brain was something similar to a massive, swarming ant colony or a huge housing project for wayward spirits with countless beings working away inside me. However, in my case, in general (certainly not always) it's more like order than disorder, and the multitude of selves who live within me appear to get along pretty well.

Comedian George Carlin once asked, "When God does acid, does he see people?" While this may make us laugh at ourselves, if we get the joke, this idea could really be hinting at a fundamental truth about who we are. When a cell in my body, which I suspect may have an individual sense of self as much as I do, has a "religious experience" and its personal boundaries blur, I think it unifies with my whole body and it would see the mind of David Jay Brown as the god that it is becoming one with. This really gets me wondering. Prior to enlightenment, does God suffer from MPD? Are we all just multiple personalities in the mind of God? As above, so below; this statement certainly rings true here when we reflect on the holographic and fractal nature of the universe.

Sometimes I think the universe is crazy, completely mad, and this realization immediately solves many mysteries about why everything is the way that it is. Living in a culture influenced by Christian theology leads people to invoke the devil when they think of God. My psychedelic experiences led me to believe that what Christians call God and the devil are merely two sides of the same entity: ourselves. There certainly does appear to be some serious darkness operating in the world, but sometimes the light and darkness are difficult to tease apart.

CORRESPONDING WITH CHARLES MANSON

In 1996 I received a two-page, single-spaced, typewritten letter from the alleged mass-murderer mastermind Charles Manson, someone I had been fascinated by since I read *Helter Skelter* as a teenager.

Wow—it was like getting a letter from the devil himself! The thoughtfully written message, with Manson's elaborate signature at the end, was a response to an interview request that I had sent him almost a year earlier, along with copies of two of my interview books. The letter was typed because, he said, "My penmanship is terrible and with age, my hands do not hold pen or pencil as easily as in the past."

What struck me most about this detailed and well-written letter was Manson's sense of ecological awareness and his message about the unity of the biosphere. He closed the letter with the following words.

Keep the Air, Trees, Water, and Animals healthy. They are the future
of the Earth, they are us, we are them, it's all one. The fires of Tara
keep burning. A.T.W.A. is life, life is A.T.W.A. Keep the belief . . .
Always . . .

Manson also praised my writing and hinted at the possibility of coauthoring a book with me. He wrote:

> I believe that the completed product may prove interesting. My rather unique philosophy, outlook, beliefs, and experiences could benefit from your experience with the written word. As an additional note, I bring to your attention that I am seriously considering authoring a book regarding the events occurring after my release from federal prison up to my conviction for the now infamous crimes. I am not getting any younger and believe it is finally time to tell "my story" of those events, which has never been told or printed. Everyone else has told their version of the story and half-truths. I am attempting to locate an author and/ or publisher who might help me in the endeavor. Do you have any suggestions as to whom I could contact in inquiry? I thank you, for your time, interest, anticipated cooperation, and any assistance you may be able to provide.

I took the bait. I was eager to get started on this unique opportunity, of course. Manson said that in order to get started I should return the California State Prison, Corcoran, visiting forms that were enclosed with his letter. However, there were no visiting forms enclosed.

So I wrote back to Manson, saying that I was interested in interviewing him and possibly writing this book with him, but there were no visiting forms enclosed. A month later I received another letter from Manson, saying:

> No, the visiting forms were not included in the previous correspondence by design. I and a friend wanted to be sure you were not playing some type of "game" which, unfortunately, I have encountered in these matters. A friend of mine will be contacting you in the near future. He has agreed to work on the legalities and

logistics and everything with you. . . . If you survive swimming with the shark, our paths shall meet again in the future. Good luck, until then . . .

Then he closed the letter with the same concluding words from his first letter.

Keep the Air, Trees, Water, and Animals healthy. They are the future of the Earth, they are us, we are them, it's all one. The fires of Tara keep burning. A.T.W.A. is life, life is A.T.W.A. Keep the belief . . . Always . . .

I received a few letters from Manson's "friend," or agent, it seemed, but, unfortunately, was never able to arrange an interview. However, I did receive those two extraordinary letters from Manson that will always mystify me. I'm fascinated by Manson's mind, and I'm intrigued by people who think differently. Timothy Leary was put in a prison cell right next to Manson at one point in his incarceration career, and in his book *Neuropolitics* he writes about Manson's nefarious use of LSD to reimprint, reprogram, and brainwash members of his cult, or "family," as religious murderers. But what intrigued me most about Manson were all his bizarre interpretations of songs by the Beatles (on the White Album) and the final chapter of the New Testament as justification for masterminding some of the most gruesome murders in recent history.

When I was in my twenties I was extremely interested in people who had psychotic tendencies and was especially compelled by the fascinating relationship between creativity and psychopathology. Working as a mental-health counselor on the acute wards of psychiatric hospitals, with people who suffered from severe psychological disorders, while doing so many psychedelic drugs sometimes made we wonder if I was going crazy. Was I? Sometimes we certainly thought so.

MY EXPERIENCE WITH SCHIZOPHRENIA, PSYCHOSIS, AND BIPOLAR DISORDER

I've long been intrigued by the relationship between creativity and psychopathology. When I interviewed Oscar Janiger he said:

> I began to look into the whole sticky issue of psychopathology and creativity. I found that there are links between the creative state and certain qualities that people say they have when they're creating, that were very much like some of the perceptions of people who were schizophrenic or insane. I began to notice what made the difference. It seemed that the artists were able to maintain a certain balance, riding the edge, as it were. I thought of creativity as a kind of dressage, riding a horse delicately with your knees. The artist was able to ride his creative Pegasus, putting little pressure on his ability to control the situation, enabling him to just master it, while allowing the rest to flow freely so that the creative spirit can take its own course. The artist is faced with the dilemma of allowing this uprush of material to enter into their conscious mind, much like trying to take a drink from a high-pressure fire hose. This allows them to integrate their technique and training, and still be able to keep relatively free of preconceived ideas, formulated notions or obligatory reality. In that state they were able to harness it enough so that the overriding symptoms of psychosis were not present, but every other aspect of their being at that time seemed as though they were in a semi-psychotic state. So I evoked the term "dry schizophrenia," where a person was able to control the surroundings and yet be "crazy" at the same time, crazy in the sense that they could use this mode of consciousness for their work and creative ability. There's a lot of documentation about psychopathology and creativity but I think it's all from a central pool, kind of a wellspring of the creative imagination that we can draw from. It equally gives its strength to psychosis in one sense, or breakthroughs in creativity, theological

revelation in the world of the near-dying, people who are seriously ill, and so on. All of that provides us with a look into this cauldron, this very dynamic, efficacious part of the brain, that for some reason or other is kept away from us by a semi-permeable membrane that could be ruptured in different ways, under different circumstances.

When I interviewed John Lilly he taught me to distinguish between insanity and "outsanity." Outsanity is consensus reality, what we all agree is real. Insanity, on the other hand, is what we privately believe to be real and that may seem crazy to others.

While few people questioned John's scientific brilliance, more than a few people questioned his sanity during some of his periods of regularly injecting ketamine. An attempted call to U.S. president Gerald Ford during one such period, to warn him about the imminent dangers of the Solid State Entities wiping out water-based life-forms on our planet, involuntarily landed the brilliant neuroscientist and renowned dolphin researcher in a New York City psychiatric hospital. However, according to Lilly, the Earth Coincidence Control Office (ECCO) intervened to save him. (John wrote me a quote for the back cover of my science-fiction novel *Virus: The Alien Strain* that utterly warmed my heart. It said, "*Virus* is fantastic. David Jay Brown is an ECCO agent.")

Despite my status as an ECCO agent, I had a number of experiences on psychedelics that personally led me to question my own sanity, and sometimes I thought that I had gone permanently insane while I was tripping—such as the first time that I did LSD as a teenager. However, I always returned from the experiences at least as sane as before I took the substance, so my concerns in this area have diminished with time.

Nonetheless, I have had my own bouts with genuine mental illness. I suffer from a mild form of what's known in psychiatric literature as rapidly cycling, bipolar II disorder, which means that my brain quickly cycles between relatively extreme emotional highs and lows, and I've had some difficulty balancing these intense emotions at times over the years. This is less severe than ordinary bipolar disorder, but the symptoms are similar and have been debilitating at times.

However, I would never choose to sacrifice my range of emotion for a stable middle ground, because I see my wide emotional range as what makes me feel alive, passionate, and creative, despite the hell that it can sometimes put me through. Psychiatric drugs, like Nardil, lithium, and SSRIs, which I've tried, put a floor and ceiling on the range of my emotional states, which not only prevents me from getting depressed but also from becoming happy—not to mention the horrifically subduing effects on my sex drive and sexual performance.

The best treatments I've found to help me keep my brain in emotional balance are cannabis, phenibut, L-tryptophan, Hydergine, L-theanine, Gerovital, and Deprenyl.

Many people have asked me if I think that all my psychedelic use has influenced my bipolar disorder, and I've thought long and hard about this. I think the answer is yes, in two primary ways. I think that it has increased the range of my emotional sensitivity, making me in some ways more vulnerable to the biochemical swings, but my experience with psychedelics has also provided me with powerful psychological skills for dealing better with the disorder, so it seems like the influences have pretty much balanced themselves out and my moods are more under control now than ever before in my life.

I have had a lot of experience with sitting up all night in psychiatric hospitals talking thoughtfully with ranting schizophrenics about their ideas. I found their minds utterly fascinating. In fact, at one hospital I was actually fired for spending too much time with the patients! I loved talking to them about their strange ideas, their unusual beliefs, and their paranoid delusions, although, for the most part, this was a population that was severely debilitated and clearly unable to even take care of themselves. So madness, insanity, psychosis, and schizophrenia are all subjects that have greatly intrigued me, largely because as disorders of the thought process they shed much light on the nature of cognition. These encounters became the basis for the psychiatric hospital scenes in my science-fiction novels.

What intrigues me the most about psychiatric disorders is that every one seems like an exaggeration of some aspect of myself, and by seeing these aspects magnified I can understand myself better. Looking through a copy of the latest *Diagnostic and Statistical Manual of Mental Disorders* (DSM), which identifies and describes all the known psychiatric disorders, makes me feel like I'm reading a book about myself at my worst. It seems like I have symptoms of just about every single one of the disorders described in the DSM-IV. However, in actuality these different forms of mental illness are exaggerations of psychological dynamics that are inherent in all human nervous systems.

When I interviewed the late psychiatrist Oscar Janiger, who treated me for my bipolar disorder and was a close personal friend, he told me:

> I recall reading that James Joyce had a daughter named Lucia who was schizophrenic. She was the sorrow of his life. Upon persuasion from Joyce's patron, both of them were brought to Carl Jung. This was against Joyce's wishes because he didn't like psychiatrists. Jung examined Lucia, then finally came in and sat down with Joyce. Joyce said to him that he thought Lucia was a greater artist and writer than he was. Can you imagine? So Jung said, "That may be true, but the two of you are like deep-sea divers. You go into the ocean, a rich, interesting, dramatic setting, with your baskets, and you fill them up with improbable creatures of the deep. The only difference between the two of you is that you can come up to the surface, and she can't."

"Basically it's like the difference between being able to swim in the ocean or drowning," I said. Janiger replied, "Right, like being caught by the waves and dashed to pieces."

This rang true with me. With the exception of some transitory delusions that I had several times on ketamine, I've had only one personal encounter with psychosis from an insider's perspective. In 1996, after experiencing a severe depression and emotional crisis due to a painful romantic breakup, I was mistakenly prescribed Zoloft, which triggered a manic and eventually psychotic reaction in me. I'm sure that the ketamine that I was also doing at the time didn't help. I became delusional and manic, didn't sleep a wink for nine consecutive nights, and have only vague recollections of what actually happened during that time, largely pieced together from what people told me. It became clear that Zoloft was contraindicated for people with bipolar disorder, but I had some extraordinary experiences during this time that were truly hallucinatory.

I would think that I was talking to someone on the phone for hours, only to suddenly realize that I didn't even have the phone in my hand, and, in fact, the phone was sitting at the other end of the room. I sometimes also thought that I was watching television only to suddenly realize that the screen had been completely dark and had never been on. Most weirdly, I remember examining a calendar for hours, being totally perplexed. I was looking at the dates without understanding what they were and trying to figure out what they meant, because I knew it had some importance. I just couldn't imagine what it was.

As we discussed in chapter 1, time is a strange concept to contemplate, and this is a subject that I've also thought about a lot and will be discussing more later. My frustrations with understanding what a calendar was and with time in general seemed like a foreshadowing of what I was to learn about the strange mysteries of time from my encounters with the late ethnobotanist Terence McKenna.

TERENCE MCKENNA AND THE END OF TIME

I got to know Terence McKenna largely through our close mutual friends Carolyn Mary Kleefeld and Nina Graboi and was granted access into his inner circle, so I got so spend a lot of intimate time with him. I also attended around a half-dozen workshops with Terence at the Esalen Institute in Big Sur during the late eighties and early nineties and used this valuable opportunity to explore his vast mind, which was well known for thinking supposedly unthinkable thoughts.

Terence was an exceptionally brilliant enthnobotanist who played—and continues to play—a vital role in influencing the psychedelic community. He was probably the best storyteller I've ever met, and the spellbinding talks that he routinely gave about his adventures in the Amazon experimenting with psychedelic plants and fungi were simply mesmerizing. His bejeweled descriptions of the DMT experiences, jaw-dropping encounters with the magic mushroom, and nonhuman botanical intelligence stand out as some of the very best and most eloquent descriptions of these seemingly ineffable phenomena ever to spring from the human mind.

Terence's theoretical model of time as a wave form, which was one of his formally developed theories, had an end point that supposedly arrived on December 21, 2012. According to Terence, what is primarily accelerating in evolution is novelty, newness, and this acceleration of novelty will reach a point of infinite density at the end of its cycle. The date that Terence chose for this end point coincided with the end of the Mayan calendar. This choice was part of the reason why the Mayan prophecy about the significance of the year 2012 snowballed into the cultural phenomenon that it has become and was perpetuated by writer Daniel Pinchbeck and others. According to Terence this is when history ends and novelty becomes infinite, although this date will already have passed by the time you're reading this book, and I suspect that the elusive Singularity will still appear to lie further on the horizon.

According to my interview with Terence's brother Dennis in 2008, Terence deliberately chose the end point of the Mayan calendar to coincide with the end point of his time wave, so it wasn't a synchronicity, as some people seem to believe or as Terence may have suggested. Perhaps Terence's model may coincide with a different time frame, if it is indeed true, as even he wasn't completely sure about the time frame that he chose to apply it to. Dennis McKenna's book *The Brotherhood of the Screaming Abyss* recounts his experiences with Terence and sheds much important light on his life and ideas.

I tend to think of Terence's timewave theory more like an elaborate painting, a piece of poetry, or a work of art, than a scientific theory. He was a brilliant storyteller, with an extraordinary imagination and astonishing use of language, but his timewave model doesn't produce clearly testable results, so it can never be truly proven or disproven. It seems so subjective when one tries to interpret it, but I understand that it also does seem to be reflecting a real aspect of nature when one studies it closely. It's strangely mysterious.

I think that Terence's model falls into the same category as other unexplained phenomena that can't be clearly determined, like crop circles and UFO sightings. As I discussed in chapter 3, there appears to be a certain class of phenomena that almost seems designed to provide compelling evidence without conclusive proof. I suspect that this is actually a deliberate attempt to reorganize the structure of our rational minds by a higher intelligence that is either teaching us or toying with us.

Terence had a lot of unusual and utterly fascinating ideas that truly deserve further scientific exploration, such as the notion that psilocybin mushroom spores arrived from outer space, that psychedelic mushrooms in the diet of early hominoids was the catalyst for our creation of language, and, as I mentioned, that novelty and time are accelerating with evolution. What's so perplexing about the thought-provoking ideas Terence described is that whenever I try to explain them to other people they inevitably sound completely ridiculous. However, with Terence's almost supernatural mastery of language, he could make the wildest and most far-flung ideas seem more than plausible, as if he were revealing the secrets of nature.

I really love Terence and miss his brilliant mind terribly. He wrote me a terrific quote for the back cover of my first book, *Brainchild,* in 1987, which made me giddy with happiness: "That our perfected selves whisper to us from the future is but one of David Jay Brown's fertile insights." Terence's second book, *The Archaic Revival,* also contained the interview I did with him, which later appeared in *Mavericks of the Mind.*

Terence McKenna was the very first person Rebecca Novick and I interviewed for *Mavericks of the Mind,* as well as the first interview that either one of us ever did. It was 1988; I was twenty-six years old and Bek was twenty-four. We drove to the Esalen Institute in Big Sur, California, where Terence was giving a workshop, and met with him late one afternoon at the Big House. We went to the top floor of the building and sat down on fluffy pillows on the rug in a circle with several other people. When we began our interview, Terence lit up a big fat joint of strong sinsemilla laced with generous amounts of hashish and passed it around.

It was a good thing Rebecca and I were properly prepared for the interview and had all of our questions written down on paper, because after just a few tokes of Terence's superpowered doobie, we were hardly able to speak and just barely managed to read our questions off the paper. The combination of being starstruck in Terence's presence and having the left circuit of my brain temporarily rendered virtually inoperable by the flood of potent cannabinoids left me with little to say beyond the questions that I slowly and dutifully read off the paper in my hands. Thank heavens for audio recorders!

Meanwhile, Terence, who smoked quite a bit more than we did, couldn't possibly have been more verbally animated and eloquently articulate. Terence was a master of language—the most compelling, silver-tongued storyteller I've ever met—and cannabis seemed to fuel his intellect and imagination. He also had a wonderful sense of humor.

Somehow we managed to get through the interview, and I was fortunate enough to be able to spend a good deal of intimate time with Terence before he died, much of it while high on copious amounts of cannabis that we smoked together, which was largely at his home in Occidental, California. I was increasingly mesmerized by his supernatural storytelling abilities and his extraordinary insights, historical knowledge, and scientific expertise, and I would listen to Terence speak for hours or sometimes literally for days on end.

Terence had an amazing ability to find words that expressed many things that most people had previously thought indescribable in human language, and this helped to inspire me to write the psychedelic sequences in my science-fiction novel, *Brainchild*. Terence had the most extraordinary adventures at the disposal of his mesmerizing storytelling abilities, from both his travels around the globe and in the hyperdimensional realms of high-dose psilocybin and DMT.

As one would expect, Terence had seen a lot and wasn't easily impressed, so I was pretty happy whenever I could help to surprise him. Once while Terence was visiting Big Sur sometime in the mid-1990s, after an Esalen workshop he led, I accompanied him, Carolyn Mary Kleefeld, and some other friends on a visit to the home of an extraordinarily talented sculptor named Edmund Kara.

Before entering Edmund's home and studio on the crest of Pfeiffer Point, I raved enthusiastically to Terence, "You're in for a real treat; these are some of the most incredible sculptures you've ever seen!"

Terence looked at me with more than just a little skepticism and a facial expression that seemed to be politely saying, "Don't you know who you're talking to?" He simply said, "We'll see."

However, after about five minutes inside Edmund's magical studio, where majestic mythological figures sprang to life, Terence turned to me and said, "I see what you mean." You can see Edmund Kara's extraordinary work at www.edmundkara.com.

Terence died of a brain tumor in 2000. The tumor was located in the right prefrontal cortex, an area primarily associated with the imagination and future speculation—the very areas where Terence seemed so especially gifted. Because these were the areas in which Terence seemed to excel, I couldn't help wondering if there might have been some connection. In the 1996 film *Phenomenon*, John Travolta plays the role of a gifted individual who develops extraordinary mental powers, psychic abilities, and even has mystical experiences, all as a result, we learn later in the film, of being caused by a brain tumor that eventually kills him. I couldn't help thinking of Terence when I saw this film.

Since Terence died I've had numerous dreams with him in them, and a number of people have told me that they have seen him during mushroom or DMT encounters. I hope he's now a happy, self-transforming machine elf somewhere in hyperspace. Although I first became familiar with Terence from a tape that someone sent me when I was attending NYU, it was my dear friend Carolyn Kleefeld who intro-duced me to Terence. Carolyn is a truly extraordinary individual, and she has had an immense influence on my life.

SINGING SONGS OF ECSTASY WITH
CAROLYN MARY KLEEFELD

I got to know poet, painter, and philosopher Carolyn Mary Kleefeld in 1983. We've remained close friends ever since, and she has had an enormous influence on my work in many ways. I am deeply in debt to her for believing so strongly in my work over the years.

I first got to know Carolyn through her poetry. I picked up a copy of her book *Lovers in Evolution* at the Bodhi Tree Bookstore in West Hollywood when I was in college at USC. I used to love to spend hours hanging out at the landmark metaphysical bookstore before working at Altered States, the isolation tank center where I trained new psy-chonauts every weekend.

I was totally blown away by Carolyn's magnificent poetry in the book, which spoke from a post-terrestrial, genetic perspective on the human condition, with humor and psychedelic insight, that I really resonated with. Timothy Leary gave her much praise at the time. It was simply a delightful find, and I treasured the book.

Several months later, after graduating from USC with a degree in psychobiology, I attended a weeklong workshop by Timothy Leary at the fabled Esalen Institute in Big Sur on the evolution of intelligence. It was Tim's very last workshop there. On my first night I met one of Carolyn's daughters, whom I soon fell in love with. While the romance with Carolyn's daughter lasted only a year, my friendship with Carolyn felt like tapping back in to an ancient, timeless connection, and we maintain it strongly to this day.

Carolyn and I have gone on endless magical adventures together through the heavenly wilderness of Big Sur and have spent years philosophizing about the creative process, the human condition, and the nature of reality. Many of my ideas have been influenced by nightlong conversations with her, and a lot of my writing projects emerged from our interactions.

Carolyn is also an extraordinarily talented and unusually unique painter whose work is exhibited worldwide in books, galleries, and museums and on websites. I've literally spent whole nights staring at just a single painting that she's done, which can sometimes became a clear portal into another universe. Her paintings truly seem like polished windows that reveal the hidden dimensions of reality. She has written a number of highly acclaimed poetry books, and an in-depth interview that I did with her can be found in my book *Mavericks of the Mind*.

Carolyn also did the cover of my first book, *Brainchild,* a fantastic painting that I deeply love called *Neuro-Erotic Blast-Off.* The book is not only dedicated to her; the main character was partially inspired by her. Carolyn also participated in the roundtable discussions that Rebecca Novick and I did with other eminent figures in the early 1990s at UCLA and UCSC. Transcripts of these discussions can be found in the second edition of *Mavericks of the Mind.*

Carolyn also did the art for the *MAPS Bulletin* about psychedelics and technology that I edited in 2008, and we have made numerous contributions to one another's works over the years. She has been one of my closest friends, and she believed in me when no one else would. Her support of my work and belief in what I'm doing has been immeasurable, and I'll be forever in her debt. You can find out more about Carolyn's inspiring books and beautiful artwork online by visiting www.carolynmarykleefeld.com.

Another person whom I also feel immeasurably indebted to is Nina Graoi, who was a close friend of Carolyn's and mine, and she also had a profound effect on my life.

ONE FOOT IN THE FUTURE AND BEYOND

I met Nina Graboi in 1987 through our mutual friend Robert Forte, another person who has had a strong influence on my life.

I met Robert, or Bob as he is usually known, at a party in the early eighties that Peter Stafford, author of *The Psychedelics Encyclopedia,* was giving in Santa Cruz. Bob and I became close friends, and he has remained one ever since. Robert is the author of *Entheogens and the Future of Religion* and *Timothy Leary: Outside Looking In.* In addition to Nina Graboi, Bob introduced me to Oscar Janiger, who also played a vital role in my life, and my discussions with Bob over the years have been engaging and enlightening.

Nina Graboi became something like a grandmother to both me and Bob, and we loved her dearly. She was a truly remarkable woman. Born in Vienna, Austria, in 1918, she fled the Nazi takeover of her country and spent three months in a detention camp in North Africa. Through a mixture of ingenuity and good fortune she managed to escape and come to America with her husband in 1941. Arriving as a penniless refugee, she went on to become a society hostess in an exclusive Long Island community. At age thirty-six she was living what most people considered the epitome of the American dream, yet Nina felt a great void in her life. In search of this missing link, she plunged into the study of esoteric subjects and became an avid practitioner of meditation. When she was forty-seven she left her husband and became deeply involved in the counterculture of the sixties.

Nina had her first psychedelic experience in the company of Alan Watts, and she frequently spent time at the famed Millbrook estate where a group had gathered around Timothy Leary to study the mind-expanding effects of LSD. She was the director of the New York center of the League for Spiritual Discovery, a nonprofit organization that operated to help and educate people engaged in exploring the potential of psychedelic consciousness, and was an active member of the Wo/Men's Alliance for Medical Marijuana (WAMM) in Santa Cruz, California.

Nina's autobiography, *One Foot in the Future,* chronicles her remarkable spiritual journey and has been described by Terence McKenna as "an extraordinary tale of humor and hope." I took the photograph of

Nina on the cover of the book on Carolyn Kleefeld's property in Big Sur on an especially magical day. An interview with Nina appears in my book *Mavericks of the Mind*.

Carolyn, Nina, and I spent a lot of time together attending workshops at Esalen and exclusive parties, and visiting with psychedelic celebrities. One of my favorite places to hang out was at the Mondo 2000 temple in the Berkeley Hills.

R.U. SIRIUS AND *MONDO 2000*

On par with *MAD* magazine and *Scientific American*, *Mondo 2000* was one of the most influential magazines I ever read. I was thrilled to watch its rapid evolution out of the psychedelic primordial ooze of earlier, more fringe incarnations, as *High Frontiers* and *Reality Hackers* and into the central role that it played in the cyberpunk culture of the 1990s.

I was simply amazed by how quickly the whole process snowballed, and a significant portion of today's mainstream digital culture, and the more radical transhumanism movement, began with *Mondo 2000*'s explorations into psychedelic science and its celebrations of the early Internet, mind-expanding technologies, and erotic paganism. Personally it was exciting evidence for me that the cultural transformations predicted by my teenage heroes Timothy Leary and Robert Anton Wilson were indeed becoming a reality. Now, of course, we're in full swing, with a psychedelic Internet culture sweeping across the globe.

I met R.U. Sirius in 1983 in *The Psychedelics Encyclopedia* author Peter Stafford's apartment at the La Bahia Hotel on Beach Street in Santa Cruz shortly after I moved to the coastal college town. R.U. showed up one afternoon while I was there and started excitedly spreading out the layout for the first issue of what was to become *High Frontiers* on the floor of Peter's living room. I was just twenty-one, and I remember being somewhat astonished that there was actually a culture here that was familiar with Timothy Leary and Robert Anton Wilson's work. I thought there were just a handful of people on the planet who knew what the eight-circuit model of the brain was or who passionately shared my optimistic longing for a psychedelic future of abundance, freedom, and magic. Everywhere that I had previously lived, I was pretty much the only one.

Although I loved the inspiring ideas behind what I was seeing on Peter's messy floor—as R.U. proudly displayed his newspaper-like creation—initially, to be honest, I thought the articles and images looked somewhat amateurish and the pro-psychedelic and pro-technology tabloid looked a bit geeky, maybe even kind of silly, so I was simply astonished by what it evolved into. It became the slick, glossy, futuristic magazine that I had been eagerly awaiting since I first tripped on acid as a teenager, and I'm sure that a lot of other people felt the same way about it, as *Mondo 2000* attracted world-class writers, artists, scientists, and thinkers. It absolutely blew my mind, and I still treasure every issue.

I loved the extraordinary *Mondo 2000* parties at their magnificent temple in the Berkeley Hills, and I had some of the most memorable times of my life at these events. I met many kindred spirits at the exclusive gatherings, people who also thought that science was sexy, psychedelics were transcendental, and nothing was cooler than discussing ideas about physical immortality, increasing our intelligence, and activating new states of consciousness. I had telepathic conversations with new friends while tripping on exotic psychedelics, and I learned a lot about virtual reality, smart drugs, and the parapsychological implications of quantum physics.

Chemists invited me to sample their latest mind-bending pharmacological creations, which was like tempting a kid in a candy store. If, after doing so, I found myself in the midst of a totally tripped-out conversation with some supercute, supersmart girl I just met there, and I had some burning question about chemistry, nanotechnology, lucid dreaming, or chaos theory, world-class experts on these fascinating subjects were all around to ask. The *Mondo 2000* parties were extraordinarily fun, and it was at these ultrahip yet geeky gatherings—where nerdy, tech-savvy Internet enthusiasts were actually considered cool—that I met many of the people who were to later become my colleagues and coconspirators in the global plot to raise the consciousness of our wayward species.

It was through interacting with this crowd that I began to sense how psychedelics could be integrated into Western society and how they were dramatically affecting the direction of our future evolution. In the next chapter we'll examine what the future evolution of our species might look like.

6
The Psychobiology of Gods and Goddesses

I think our entire evolutionary history is recorded in our genetic code and that it is available for us to review in the appropriate state of consciousness. Additionally, I suspect that the future stages of our evolution are also already encoded in our DNA, the same way that an acorn contains an oak tree, and that we can glimpse previews of our future evolutionary stages while on high doses of psychedelics. The first stage of psychedelic development involves healing from our inevitable, earlier wounds.

THE HEALING POTENTIAL OF PSYCHEDELICS, AND MIND-BODY MEDICINE

When I was in college during the early eighties, my maverick mentor, alternative physician Russell Jaffe told me that the most effective tool discovered by modern medicine was being overlooked by the majority of physicians. Jaffe was referring to the placebo effect, the power of the mind to affect the health of the body. Numerous studies have demonstrated that what we believe about a medical treatment dramatically affects how we respond to it. This is why when pharmaceutical companies develop a new drug it is always tested against inactive sugar pills—placebos—that are known to improve symptoms and facilitate cures simply because the patient and/or the physician believes that the new drug might work.

Ironically, when I studied psychobiology at USC and NYU, I was taught by most of my professors that the placebo effect was simply something to be controlled for in experimental or clinical trials. In other words, it was a nuisance that interfered with our understanding of the effects of a new drug or procedure, and most researchers and health care practitioners simply shrugged off the placebo effect as simply irrelevant. This was in the days before we really understood that what we believe not only directly impacts how we feel, but it measurably affects our physiology as well. We now know that the mind and body are simply two parts of the same inseparable system, and each dramatically affects the other.

Candace Pert, the neuroscience researcher who discovered the opiate receptor in the brain (and whom I interviewed for my previous book, *Conversations on the Edge of the Apocalypse*), brought about a paradigm shift in modern medicine by pioneering research that revealed an intimate relationship between the mind and body. Her interdisciplinary research into the relationship between the nervous system and the immune system demonstrated a body-wide communication system mediated by peptide molecules and their receptors. Pert believes this to be the biochemical basis of emotion and the potential key to understanding many challenging diseases. Pert's research provides a basis for understanding why cancer patients can measurably reduce tumor growth through the process of visualization and why placebos can cause measurable physiological changes.

In his practice as a general and pediatric surgeon, Bernie Siegel began recognizing common personality characteristics in patients who did well and those who didn't. In his bestselling book *Love, Medicine, and Miracles,* Siegel describes how exceptional cancer patients survive because of their attitude and beliefs. When I spoke with Siegel he told me, "You can't separate thoughts and beliefs from your body. In other words, what you think, and what you believe, literally change your body chemistry."

Studies confirm Siegel's observations. For example, a PET-scan study conducted at the University of Michigan showed that people who believed they were receiving a painkiller actually produced more pain-killing endorphins in their brains and experienced less pain.

A relatively recent branch of medicine known as mind-body medicine addresses this fascinating and important topic. When I wrote *Mavericks of Medicine,* I spoke with Bernie Siegel, Andrew Weil, and Larry Dossey about how we might be able to use this understanding to improve our health. I also spoke with psychopharmacology researchers Raphael Mechoulam and Rick Strassman about the therapeutic potential of cannabis and psychedelic drugs. Many hallucinogenic plants—such as peyote and ayahausca brews—have a long history of shamanic and medicinal use in healing practices around the world, and they may enhance the strength of the placebo effect (i.e., the power of the mind) because of their consciousness-changing abilities.

When I interviewed Weil he told me about how he had become completely cured of a lifelong cat allergy during an LSD session when he was twenty-eight and that this experience had a profound influence on his medical perspective, which we'll be discussing more in chapter 7. Weil's experience is a good example of how psychedelics may act as placebo-effect amplifiers, and this idea may be the key to understanding the great medical value they have, because one of the primary aspects of the mind that psychedelics act upon is our sense of *belief.* In other words, the enormous healing power of psychedelics may lie in their extraordinary ability to affect what we actually believe to be true about reality and ourselves.

Ayahuasca-based shamanism has been widely reported to help heal people from a variety of difficult-to-treat illnesses. Although the body's innate ability to heal itself from illness is often brushed aside in medical research trials as *merely* the placebo effect, with ayahuasca-based shamanism the body's innate healing ability takes center stage.

In ayahuasca ceremonies it seems that the power of the mind to affect the body becomes greatly magnified, and there are numerous, well-documented stories of people who have had both long-standing medical illnesses suddenly and miraculously vanish or vastly improve after an ayahuasca healing session.

I've heard that in South America many traditional shamans who use ayahuasca in their healing ceremonies will sometimes mix some sleight-of-hand magic with real healing work, because it helps to create a state of suspended belief and a shift in awareness that ultimately affects one's belief about what is real and possible. When I spoke with the celebrated stage magician and shamanism expert Jeff McBride, I asked him if he had any thoughts about the healing potential of suspended disbelief and how it might relate to what is known about the placebo effect in modern medicine. He said:

> These shamanic healers are sometime called "sucking doctors." One of the old shamanic techniques was that the shaman would put his mouth on the affected area and suck. Then he would spit out all kinds of weird bits of bones, bugs, twisted tumor, and things like that to, I guess, create a placebo effect. Now, in the magical belief system, or ritual contract of these healing seances, that's fair game. And that has changed into what's called psychic surgery. South America and the Philippines are famous for their psychic surgeons. Sleight-of-hand magicians have a different take on this. People like James Randi and the other debunkers and skeptics see these shamans as con artists. I see it a bit differently. I think that, yes, I would say that 80 to 90 percent of them are using sleight-of-hand technique. But given the culture and the surrounding mind-set and group belief system that these "healings" are taking place in, they can possibly result in a placebo effect, which leads to a genuine cure. That's very different from what I do at ritual theater. When I pull a beam of light from my heart and I place it on your heart, I do not expect you to believe that I

have tapped in to the cosmic force of nature and am able to pull a light beam from my heart and place it in your heart. It's a way of connecting with you through a magical illusion. What this does is it creates a symbol, and a metaphor, for us sharing light from our heart with each other. Now, I can do that very same thing at a magic show in Las Vegas, and people will go, "How did you do that?" At a ritual, when I offer this light from my heart to a person that I may have had conflict with, and I take it out and I place it in their heart, then they'll say, "I'm so glad you did that," and not even think of the how. There are ways of using magic in symbol and metaphor that can create an altered state of consciousness. And in that moment of altered consciousness, a profound psychic experience can occur that influences how we frame the way we live and work in the world.

When combined with a psychedelic experience, a shift in belief created by the placebo effect can have powerful real-world consequences, and I suspect that there may be a wealth of medical value in researching this possibility.

I participated in a traditional Native American Church peyote ceremony when I was in my midtwenties, and many of the people were there for a healing of some sort. There were countless stories being told about how the peyote spirit, Mescalito, had healed people of illnesses and addictions. Personally, I found having to sit up straight in a tepee for twelve hours while I was tripping and nauseous to be more than a bit tiring, which is why I've been reluctant to journey in traditional ayahuasca circles. The night I did peyote with the Native Americans after tripping for seven hours I wanted so badly to just stretch out and relax at around four in the morning, but the shaman leading the ceremony kept scolding me like I was a misbehaving grade-school student every time I began to slouch. The participants sat in a circle around a fire and sang traditional songs all night, and some professed to miraculous healings. However, for me the most exciting

part of the night came when I witnessed a giant green goddess strad-
dling the tepee, taking all of us inside of her giant yoni as rivers of her
red menstrual blood flowed fluidly through the tepee.

Ayahuasca, peyote, and magic mushrooms are well known as potential healing agents and are worthy of more medical research. There have
been some important anthropological studies, by Dennis McKenna,
Luis Eduardo Luna, Marlene Dobkin de Rios, Barbara Myerhoff, and
others, on shamanism that incorporates these psychedelic plants and
fungi and that suggest enormous value. However, less known as a psychedelic healing agent is the strange Central American sage mint known
as *Salvia divinorum,* which I have found to be a fascinating botanical
wonder.

DJB MEETS SALVIA

Within around thirty seconds of smoking the dark herbal extract
the effects rapidly began, and I felt my entire sense of identity suddenly shift. I was instantly transformed from a human being into a
tiny disembodied speck of consciousness, completely bewildered as to
what I was and amnesic of my former identity. I was suspended in a
hyperspatial dimension, a vast crystalline communication network of
pulsing energies that was filled with countless other miniature beings
like me.

I found myself inside a kind of hidden space within space that
appeared to transcend the whole three-dimensional universe. Suddenly
my identity shifted again as a portion of the space and beings around
me folded and twisted into me, becoming a part of me. More and
more layers of the space around me continued folding into me, with
a clickety-click motion, and these layers of miniature beings became
a part of my now expanding sense of identity, until, finally, I was my
familiar human self again.

ADVENTURES WITH MAZATEC MINT

Although the Latin name for Mexican sage, *Salvia divinorum,* literally translates as "sage of the seers," this powerful hallucinogenic plant goes by a number of other names, such as Shka Pastora ("Leaves of the Shepherdess"), Diviner's Sage, ska María Pastora, yerba de Maria, Magic Mint, Sally-D, and salvia. Until fairly recently this innocent-looking member of the Mint family—whose hallucinogenic powers can dwarf those of magic mushrooms and LSD—was virtually unknown outside of a small region of Central Mexico, where it has been used as a shamanic healing tool by the Mazatec Indians in Oaxaca for at least hundreds of years. The Mazatec shamans use salvia to facilitate divinatory or visionary states of consciousness during their spiritual healing sessions when psilocybin mushrooms aren't in season.

According to my interview with ethnobotanist Daniel Siebert:

The Mazatec shamans primarily take it ceremonially as a tool for gaining access to the supernatural world or what they believe to be the realm of divine beings and supernatural entities.

Salvia divinorum is a sprawling perennial herb found in moist, isolated, and shaded regions of Oaxaca, where it grows to well over a meter in height. Salvia has hollow, square stems; large, green leaves; and occasional white and purple flowers but only rarely produces viable seed. There's nothing particularly striking about the way that this plant looks, and it easily blends in with ordinary houseplants. Like corn and bananas, salvia is thought to be a cultigen. This means that it is not known to grow in the wild. It may have been bred in cultivation, or it may have grown wild in Central Mexico at one time. Salvia leaves contain the extremely potent dissociative psychedelic compound salvinorin A.

Salvia has had a relatively hidden existence for most of its history and was known only to the Mazetec Indians and a small handful of anthropologists who were dubious about its psychoactive properties. However, since the mid-1990s it has been widely available in the United States, Europe, and other parts of the globe, largely as a smokable herb. Salvia's popularity is primarily due to the discussion of its psychoactive properties on the Internet and improved methods of ingestion that have been developed, as well as vendors promoting its sale as a legal halluci-nogen online, where many businesses sell live *Salvia divinorum* plants, dried leaves, extracts, and other preparations.

Terence McKenna was one of the first Westerners, in the mid-1990s, to publicly discuss salvia's strange hallucinogenic effects, not long after Siebert discovered the psychoactive properties of salvinorin A in 1993, as well as the proper methods for ingesting it to obtain hallucinogenic effects. Salvinorin A does not appear to be active when eaten, and it may be destroyed in the digestive system, but it can be smoked or absorbed sublingually through the mucous membranes of the mouth.

Salvia's current popularity is also a bit mysterious, because so many people find its effects unpleasant. Everyone who tries salvia agrees: this is definitely no party drug, and a large percentage of peo-ple, it seems, have no interest in even trying it a second time. "Only a small percentage of people actually buy it more than once. It's not fun in the way people normally seek out drugs," said Rick Doblin, director of MAPS. According to Brian D. Arthur, who founded the online herbal supply company Mazatec Garden, there are few repeat customers for his salvia products, "maybe 20 percent or less; most are new customers."

Arthur thinks that salvia's current popularity isn't mysterious at all; he thinks it's due to all the mainstream-media stories about it, which supports my theory that genetic intelligence helps to outlaw psychedel-ics in order to spread the word about them. He said:

> Salvia's popularity is primarily due to the constant barrage of sensa-tionalist media stories. *The New York Times, The LA Times, USA*

Today, The Today Show, Dr. Phil, and *The Doctors* have all promi-nently featured salvia. Salvia has been regularly featured by the media since 2001 as a "dangerous new Internet drug." Every time a mainstream article comes out, sales skyrocket.

Salvia is considered by most who use it to be a serious shamanic tool. Unlike LSD, magic mushrooms, or cannabis, even mild salvia journeys are far too otherworldly to be used in a social context. YouTube is filled with disturbing videos of reckless teenagers smoking salvia for the first time, then spacing out and acting weird and disoriented for about five minutes while their friends laugh and tease them. The Mazatec sha-mans would be seriously appalled, I'm sure, but this type of careless use also concerns respectful psychonauts and research scientists not only because these people may be endangering themselves but also because they are placing the plant's legal status in jeopardy.

Salvia's legal status varies considerably from country to country, and within the United States it varies from state to state. In the past few years a number of states have either made salvia illegal or have restricted its sale to adults over the age of eighteen, yet it remains precariously unscheduled in the United States on a federal level—although the Drug Enforcement Administration is closely monitoring it and is considering listing it as a controlled substance. To stay up-to-date on salvia's legal status around the world see www.sagewisdom .org/legalstatus.html.

SALVIA'S POSSIBLE MEDICAL APPLICATIONS

Some scientific researchers are concerned that legal restrictions on salvia, or its primary psychoactive component, salvinorin A, will pre-vent them from being able to easily study the plant's possible medical properties, while doing little or nothing to prevent misuse of the plant by young people, as has happened in the past with other psychedelics. Salvinorin A is unique among psychedelic substances in how it targets the brain, which could make the plant or its derivative chemicals useful for treating a number of different medical conditions.

Pharmacologically speaking, salvinorin A appears to be a relatively safe compound. No one has ever suffered a life-threatening pharmacological reaction from it, and no long-term negative physical effects have been observed. According to pharmacologist Oliver Grundmann and colleagues at the University of Florida, animal studies with salvinorin A demonstrate a lack of evidence of any short- or long-term toxicity, and the Mazetec Indians have used it safely for many generations. Salvinorin A has unique psychoactive properties and unusual neurochemical activity in the brain, which has led a number of scientific researchers to speculate that it may have valuable medical properties and applications.

Doblin said that legal restrictions on salvinorin A could make future research and clinical studies with the drug much more difficult. This would be unfortunate, because a number of researchers think that salvinorin A, or its chemical analogs, may have possible applications not only as an antidepressant but also as an analgesic and as a therapeutic tool for treating stimulant-drug addictions, some types of stroke, and Alzheimer's disease.

The painkilling properties of salvinorin A and its analogs have been studied by Tom Prisinzano, a medicinal chemist at the University of Kansas, and Bruce Cohen at Harvard Medical School has been developing chemical analogs of salvinorin A for their possible antidepressant and mood-modulation properties. Bryan Roth and colleagues at the University of North Carolina think that salvinorin A shows promise in providing new insights into the working of the brain, drug dependence, and psychosis.

Many people who have tried salvia report an improved mood afterward, and this lasting antidepressant effect may offer a new route of treatment for clinical depression. In one survey published on Erowid, Matthew Baggott found that 44.8 percent of salvia users reported an improved mood afterward, and 25.8 percent experienced antidepressant-like effects lasting twenty-four hours or more after use. Other commonly reported aftereffects include an increased feeling of insight, a sense of calmness, and an increased sense of connection with nature.

Siebert and a number of researchers think that salvinorin A's unique pharmacological properties may lead to new types of pain medications, and a number of pharmacologists are currently trying to create chemical analogs of salvinorin A that have pain-relieving or antidepressant properties without mind-bending psychedelic effects. However, some psychotherapists think that salvinorin A's consciousness-altering effects may also have useful medical applications and that the unusual states of mind that it engenders may have the potential to enhance certain forms of psychotherapy. A number of different psychedelic drugs are currently being studied to assess their ability to enhance the psychotherapeutic process and help people suffering from difficult-to-treat psychiatric disorders. Siebert and others think salvinorin A's hallucinogenic properties might be useful in this regard as well.

As was determined by Bryan Roth and colleagues in 2002 at the National Institute of Mental Health, salvinorin A is an organic chemical called a diterpenoid, which is a potent k-opioid (kappa-opioid) receptor agonist in the brain—it binds to a specific type of opiate receptor in the brain but does not activate the mu-opioid receptor that morphine acts on, which makes morphine euphoric and addictive.

Unlike the actions of the "classical" psychedelics, salvinorin A has no actions at the serotonin 2A receptor—which is the principal molecular target responsible for the psychedelic effects of LSD, psilocybin, DMT, and mescaline—and it is the first nonalkaloid psychedelic ever discovered. Salvinorin A also has effects that are nothing like the traditional opiates, and it is the most potent natural psychedelic known. Like LSD, salvinorin A is active in the microgram dosage range; a few hundred micrograms—a mere speck, the size of a very small grain of salt—is enough to launch most people into the far reaches of hyperspace.

Although the traditional use of salvia by the Mazatec Indians in Oaxaca involves chewing the leaves, most Westerners smoke them. Smoking dried salvia leaves in their natural state is often ineffective, because the plant doesn't produce salvinorin A in very large quantities. Because of this extracts are made of the leaf, which are then reapplied to the leaf to increase its potency.

These extracts vary in potency from around five to a hundred times the average amount of naturally occurring salvinorin A, and the resulting grades of salvia leaf are usually referred to by a number followed by an x, such as 5x, 10x, and so forth. This is generally indicative of the relative amounts of leaf used in preparation, but reports seem to indicate that they vary considerably in consistency. Although the numbers may be roughly indicative of the relative concentration of salvinorin A, the measure should not be taken as absolute. Potency will depend on the naturally varying strength of the untreated leaf used in preparing the extract and the efficiency of the extraction process.

WHAT DOES AN EXPERIENCE WITH SALVIA FEEL LIKE?

When smoked salvia is often reported to produce an experience relatively brief in duration, with the peak rarely lasting more than five or ten minutes, although subjectively this may feel much longer. The experience usually begins around thirty seconds after holding the smoke in one's lungs, and one is completely back to baseline after around thirty or forty minutes.

Chewing on a quid of rolled salvia leaves, as the Mazatec shamans do, or allowing an alcohol-based herbal tincture of the plant to soak in one's mouth under the tongue for around fifteen minutes produces a different type of experience than smoking it. The effects come on gradually over a period of fifteen minutes, are gentler, and last significantly longer— generally for a full hour or two. People disagree as to whether smoking or sublingual absorption is preferable. In my personal experiments with the substance, I far preferred the sublingual tincture. I found the experience much easier to work with, and it's a gentler ride. However, others prefer the rapid onset, brief duration, and greater intensity that come with smoking it.

While under the influence of salvia people often report radical shifts in perception, seeing visions with their eyes closed, and seeing visual changes with eyes open. Sometimes people find themselves laughing uncontrollably, even though they don't find anything to be particularly funny. Time and space can become distorted in strange ways. The sensation of being pushed, pulled, twisted, or taken into alternative dimensions and other realities is common, as is the feeling of other presences, other people, and nonhuman-entity contact. The plant itself is often perceived as a female spirit while under its influence.

Higher doses can cause people to completely dissociate from their body, and people who ingest strong doses need to be watched carefully so that they don't accidentally harm themselves. With higher doses, sometimes people get up and walk around, completely oblivious to their physical surroundings, and start bumping into furniture and walls. I saw one YouTube video where someone fell out a window after smoking salvia, and it didn't look fake. Experienced salvia users insist that a sober sitter always be present when one is experimenting with the plant.

With strong doses of salvinorin A all thinking in the brain shuts down, although a very lucid awareness remains and people become completely immersed in another world. Often people completely forget that they are under the influence of a psychoactive substance. After the experience ends many people describe feeling an "afterglow," an upbeat, life-affirming antidepressant effect that lasts for around a day or more.

However, many people find the effects of salvia to be unpleasant, and some people have had extremely frightening reactions to it. People can experience states of terror and panic, perhaps more so than with other, gentler psychedelics, such as LSD or magic mushrooms. Although subjectively altogether different, the effects of salvinorin A are comparable to the superpsychedelic intensity of DMT. Smoking strong doses of salvia can be psychologically unsettling if one isn't properly prepared—and even if one is. Psychonauts repeatedly stress that this substance is a powerful shamanic tool and is not for psychedelic novices. Some people have had extremely frightening, utterly hellish experiences with salvia that shook them up for weeks or months afterward.

Another common experience with salvia, which relates to my discussion about lucid dreaming, is that things we normally perceive as inanimate objects appear to be made up of conscious beings or spirits. Like the furniture in the background of Disney films, clocks, toys, and lamps take on personalities, and many people actually feel like they become inanimate objects, such as a chair, a table, or the varnish on a piece of furniture.

The late author D. M. Turner describes becoming the side of a house after smoking salvinorin A, and he was concerned he would stay that way forever. Some experiences can be even more bizarre. One person wrote about an experience where she relived a memory from her early childhood when she was playing with a cherished toy, only she reexperienced the memory from the point of view of the toy. Another person wrote to me saying that she became the couch in the house where her mother grew up, and—from the furniture's perspective—watched her mother as a child and then as a teenager and gained insight into why her mother valued conformity so much.

Because experiences with salvia can seem so strange and alien, some people have considerable difficulty integrating it into their personal lives, or even relating to it as a human being. One person on Erowid wrote, "Whatever it was I was falling into, or becoming, or being snatched up in, it had some vague connection with humanity—but it was like humanity was one small node in its superstructure." To some people the trip is largely incomprehensible. I'm reminded of a young woman I watched smoking salvia on YouTube. As she came back from a particularly harrowing journey, she simply repeated, "What the fuck just happened? What the fuck just happened?"

When I first became interested in salvia I started several discussions about the magical herb on Tribe.net. In one of the discussions Stuart wrote:

The experience of *Salvia divinorum* doesn't compare to any other entheogen. It's more like . . . everything in your life experience is images projected on a screen, a screen so omnipresent that you'd never noticed it, and now the screen gets shredded to bits. I couldn't say it's a good thing or a bad thing. But it's a WOW thing, to the greatest degree. If I were to offer it to a friend, I'd make very very sure that the friend understood that one should try this only if one highly highly values WOW experiences.

Another person wrote to me with the following words, which, I think, express the views of a lot of people who build up a relationship with salvia and integrate it successfully into their lives.

The majority of salvia aficionados have a sacred intention. According to . . . [Matthew Baggott's] survey on Erowid, seventy-four percent of repeat visitors do so for reasons described as spiritual. . . . I think that the overwhelming impression is that this is sacred . . . and not to be trifled with . . . a profound mystical portal of deep and bewildering significance that can bestow peace, healing, gratitude, and wonder.

Again and again, the most common response I got from regular salvia users was that they used it as part of a spiritual practice, which echoes the original intention of the Mazetec shamans. J. D. Arthur explains why this is so in his fascinating book *Peopled Darkness*. Arthur writes, "Salvia can restore, if only for a few moments, our birthright of pure thoughtless awareness that lies quietly beneath the clatter of thought." What Arthur is describing appears to dovetail with the goal of many Eastern spiritual practices, such as Buddhism and Hinduism.

My experience with psychedelics, especially *Salvia divinorum,* has largely convinced me that everything, including what we believe to be inanimate objects, is conscious, intelligent, and aware. One is never alone, and everything is alive. We are always surrounded by a choir of animate spirits, watching and interacting with us on subtle levels of which we're barely aware.

I had this intuition as a child that everything around me was alive. Toys, trees, buildings, cars, sidewalks—all had an intelligent presence to me as a young child. I had forgotten about this until I started experimenting with saliva, which instantly reminded me that everything is conscious, everything has a unique personality, and this conviction isn't easily shaken off.

I think most human beings suffer from some degree of autism, the inability to recognize and socially connect with other people's minds. Or, rather, autism is an exaggerated form of the mechanism in human beings that perceptually blinds us from easily recognizing how pervasive consciousness is outside the limitations of our own minds. I think that salvia helps to correct this blindness in human beings and help them realize that everything is conscious to some degree.

Every time I've done salvia the experience has been different and indescribably weird. One recent time I smoked it I had one of the strangest experiences I've ever had with the sacred plant. A few seconds after smoking the salvia, of course, I totally forgot that I smoked it. I was still in the room with my friend, except this giant conveyer belt was now traveling in a huge loop around the whole room, and I was slowly getting caught up in it and pulled along.

The conveyer belt went forward directly ahead of me, then went up the wall in front of me, turned at the ceiling back toward my direction, and then turned again at the wall and came down again toward me, dragging me along with it. I remembered where I was and who I was with, but I couldn't figure out what was happening. I heard my friend saying that everything was okay, but I wanted to say, *What do you mean? I'm totally getting caught in this crazy conveyer belt!* It took me a few minutes before I could figure out what was happening.

The visions or imagery I see behind closed eyes while tripping on salvia appear to move and transform at a certain speed, and the bizarre organic forms and alien landscapes that I tend to see change with mental "clicks" that last about a second each. The interesting thing about the salvia-inspired imagery is that as each transformation occurs what is perceived as figure and what is perceived as ground keep shifting in my field of vision. After reflecting upon these strange visions it occurred to me that this is how a hyperdimensional object or a multidimensional landscape might appear from the limited, three-dimensional perspective of a human being.

A lot of people describe their experiences with salvia and DMT as being akin to entering a higher dimension, and this makes a lot of sense to me. Physicist Michio Kaku's book *Hyperspace: A Scientific Odyssey through Parallel Universes, Time Warps, and the Tenth Dimension* and Rob Bryanton's *Imagining the Tenth Dimension* both seem to provide uncanny maps of the territory that one encounters after smoking salvia or DMT. Like the two-dimensional characters in Edwin Abbott's book *Flatland,* we seem just as limited in our three-dimensional perspective. From a three-dimensional point of view it seems like there aren't any other directions to go besides backward and forward, right and left, up and down. But there is another direction that we can move into, another dimension that contains this one within it, and the way to get there is by going directly into the center of our own minds.

Kaku is one of my favorite science writers, and his ideas about multiple universes existing within a larger multiverse may help to explain why there are two basic types of creation myths in the world. Some people believe that the universe had a beginning and that it will have an ending, while others believe that the universe is eternal and timeless. Kaku proposes that within the eternal, timeless multiverse, new universes with finite time lines are continually being born and dying. If this is true, then it helps to explain the mystery behind our creation myths as well as where our consciousness might actually go when we smoke salvia.

LEARNING MORE ABOUT SALVIA

Several exceptionally good books, or travelogues, have been written about salvia's unusual effects. The late psychonaut D. M. Turner wrote *Salvinorin: The Psychedelic Essence of Salvia Divinorum,* which chronicles his courageous explorations with this strange botanical wonder and the synergistic combinations that he tried, mixing salvinorin A with other psychedelics. Turner's extraordinary description of the salvia spirit ferociously battling it out with the DMT spirit, like they were giant mythological titans, is worth the price of the book.

J. D. Arthur's *Peopled Darkness: Perceptual Transformation through Salvia Divinorum,* which I mentioned above, provides an unusually articulate description of salvia's seemingly indescribable effects and a fascinating discussion about how its effects can radically transform one's perception of reality over time. Martin Ball has also written an excellent book called *Sage Spirit: Salvia Divinorum and the Entheogenic Experience,* and Daniel Siebert is currently completing the definitive book on the subject.

Because salvia experiences can be so visually dramatic, its use has also inspired some pretty incredible artwork. For example, artist Luke Brown has done some especially good paintings that seem to capture some visual aspects of the salvia experience.

Hands down, the best source for scientifically accurate information about salvia and salvinorin A is Daniel Siebert's *Salvia divinorum* Research and Information Center website, www.sagewisdom.org, and his FAQ page and User's Guide are essential reading for anyone considering trying *Salvia divinorum.* Siebert also has a free e-mail newsletter called *The Salvia divinorum Observer,* which you can sign up for and which covers new scientific findings, pending legislation and changes in legal status, recent media coverage, and other updates about salvia. The *Salvia divinorum* section on Erowid is also an invaluable source of information on this fascinating plant, and the psychonaut and *Salvia divinorum* tribes on Tribe.net are lively places for discussion on the topic.

Could experiences with salvia, as well as other dimensional-shifting psychedelics and lucid dreaming, be preparing us for the realities that advanced nanotechnology will make available to us in the near future? I suspect so. I also think that combining different psychedelic compounds opens up entirely new possibilities for exploring consciousness and that these integrations may be at the forefront of the evolutionarily developed states of consciousness that lie in our near future.

I've had some of my most memorable, jaw-dropping, and valuable learning experiences with combinations of ayahuasca, LSD, magic mushrooms, *Salvia divinorum,* MDMA, and nitrous oxide. Some of my most intensely rewarding experiences came from combining different substances that had a synergistic effect. The two most synergistic psychedelics that I've found, and that go with every other psychedelic that I've tried, are cannabis and nitrous oxide.

DJB MEETS N_2O

I was a strange kid. As a child I always loved visiting the dentist. Nestled in those big, comfy, overstuffed chairs, surrounded by strange whizzing and gurgling medical instruments, I would always deeply enjoy my experience with the analgesic gas nitrous oxide (N_2O), otherwise known as laughing gas.

While my teeth were being drilled and cavities were being filled I would pleasantly drift into a dreamlike world of magical visions and enchanted cartoon landscapes. To this day I always ask for nitrous oxide whenever I go to the dentist, even if I'm just having my teeth cleaned. I often have experiences with this breathable painkiller that seem infused with mystical revelations and profound insights into the nature of reality.

Many of my early experiences with LSD as a teenager were augmented by the combined use of cannabis and nitrous oxide, and I don't think that the experiences would have been nearly as transcendent, mystical, insightful, and revelatory without these synergistic aids. I was excited to discover that the gas I loved so much at the dentist was available at my local mall or head shop, where I could purchase whipped-cream chargers, metal "crackers" to open them with, and balloons. I would do nitrous oxide balloons while on LSD and experience powerful spiritual revelations about the nature of life and death. I later began combining nitrous oxide with many other psychedelics.

UP, UP, AND AWAY IN MY GIGGLY BALLOON

Nitrous oxide is a simple gaseous compound composed of two atoms of nitrogen and one atom of oxygen: N_2O. It was first synthesized by British chemist Joseph Priestley in 1772, and pharmacologically it is classified as a dissociative anesthetic. It has been approved by the U.S. Food and Drug Administration as a safe anesthetic.

As long as inhalations of nitrous oxide are mixed with oxygen, the gas appears to be fairly safe. Suffocation from improper use and unexpectedly falling down from a lack of balance are the two greatest dangers of inhaling nitrous oxide. However, if it is only inhaled from a balloon while lying down, there appears to be little risk. According to dissociative-anesthetic expert Karl Jansen, M.D., "The urge to write philosophical tracts is probably the most serious side effect of nitrous oxide."

In the late 1700s, after his first experience with nitrous oxide, the poet Robert Southey remarked, "The atmosphere of the highest heaven must be composed of this gas." While Southey was, of course, referring to the sublimely euphoric and insight-generating properties of the gas, we now know that his statement is literally true. Nitrous oxide is the main naturally occurring regulator of stratospheric ozone in our upper atmosphere.

Southey's description of nitrous oxide is not only scientifically accurate but also poetically describes its effects quite well. Although the nitrous oxide experience lasts for only as long as one is breathing the gas, it produces a blissful feeling of escalating euphoria with repeated inhalations that build up in a manner similar to sexual arousal or a religious experience.

The gas is widely used for its ability to enhance the effects of music, because of its ability to distort and elongate the perception of sound waves, but its effects can be far more profound. The peak of a nitrous oxide experience is extremely pleasurable—reminiscent of a sexual orgasm—and it is often accompanied by a mystical sense of revelation, insight, and ecstasy. People often believe with absolute assurance that they have grasped the ultimate truth about the nature of reality, only to have this grand insight dissolve from their minds within minutes after they stop breathing the gas.

Not everyone is aware that this giggly psychedelic gas is readily and legally available for purchase outside their dentist's office at kitchen-supply stores, head shops, sex shops, online, and even at every single supermarket, because it's the only gas that's used to make whipped cream. In addition to being the propellant in whipped-cream containers, small steel cartridges containing a compressed form of the gas are sold for personal whipped-cream makers. They are commonly known as "whippets." Although these products are legally sold only to fluff up whipped cream, for many years people have been filling large balloons with them and inhaling the euphoric, mind-expanding contents.

How safe is this? The nitrous oxide that is sold for making whipped cream is categorized as food grade, which is a lower level of purity than medical grade, so it's not quite as clean as the gas that dental patients get with their root canal. I don't know of any medical studies that have been done on the health effects of inhaling food-grade nitrous oxide, but Erowid did a small study several years ago examining its effects on a filtering system. They found that a small amount of petroleum is ejected with the gas from each food-grade nitrous oxide cartridge and that a simple piece of cloth over the nozzle of the whipped cream maker seemed to filter out most of the petroleum.

There is a wonderful book on the subject called *Laughing Gas:*

Nitrous Oxide, edited by Michael Sheldin and David Wallechinsky with illustrations by Robert Crumb. To find out more about nitrous oxide see www.erowid.org/chemicals/nitrous/nitrous.shtml.

SYNERGISTIC PSYCHEDELIC COMBINATIONS

I've found that nitrous oxide goes extremely well with just about all other psychedelics, especially LSD, MDMA, and MXE.

MDMA (3,4-methylenedioxy-N-methylamphetamine) tends to amplify tactile sensations and enhance positive emotions. It generally makes people feel more empathic, more loving, more insightful, more open-minded, less fearful, and generally happier for several hours. It tends to reduce social inhibitions without diminishing clarity of thought or impairing judgment and has great psychotherapeutic potential for treating post-traumatic stress disorder, as MAPS research has demonstrated. It may also be helpful in treating autism and other psychiatric disorders. MDMA is a mild stimulant that really grounds one in the body.

As I mentioned, nitrous oxide also tends to make people feel more insightful, imaginative, and highly euphoric, although in a dissociative and highly relaxing, almost sedating, sort of way, for as long as one is breathing it. Combining these two substances can be unusually euphoric, revelatory, insightful, and fun. In Leary-Wilson terminology, it exquisitely combines the fourth, fifth, and sixth circuits.

I've had some remarkable experiences doing this extraordinary psychopharmacological combination with girlfriends, where we just sweetly cuddled and listened to music together for hours in pure heavenly bliss while being showered with rippling rainbow revelations. Cuddling on MDMA and sharing balloons of nitrous oxide with people I love have been among the most beautiful experiences of my life. Boundaries completely blur, indistinguishably dissolve, and melt together. Where one person ends and the other person begins become virtually impossible to discern. Sharing this type of experience with a loved one can be immensely pleasurable and immeasurably deepen the bond beyond what you may have thought to be previously possible.

Besides MDMA and nitrous oxide, another synergistic combination that I found to be particularly incredible was DMT and harmaline—otherwise known as ayahuasca—which I discussed earlier. These chemical matches appear to be marriages made in heaven. Adding LSD and nitrous oxide to the DMT-harmaline mix makes this combination even more amazing and more pleasant. Using nitrous oxide and LSD with harmaline and smoked DMT seems like a much more pleasant way of experiencing the benefits of ayahuasca without all the nausea, diarrhea, and purging.

Some people believe that the purging is a necessary part of the healing ayahuasca experience, although I tend to think this is largely a rationalization and is not always necessary. I think the DMT experience, by its nature, makes everything so much more meaningful, and everything that happens is so seamlessly integrated into the experience that of course it would appear that the purging is necessary, and for some people it may be. However, for people who would rather avoid this, there is another way.

Another synergistic combination that I've found to be particularly fascinating is MXE (methoxetamine) and nitrous oxide. MXE is a chemical analog of ketamine, with many of the same psychoactive properties, except that it's more potent and longer lasting. There have been no scientific studies done with MXE at the time of this writing, as it was specially developed by an underground chemist for gray-market distribution. MXE lasts almost four times longer (three hours) than ketamine, and it is about twice as strong, making it practical to snort rather than intramuscularly inject.

Intramuscular injection is often necessary with ketamine in order to get a strong enough dose to produce an out-of-body experience, a lucid dream–like state that many people describe as going into the "K hole." It also seems to be easier to remember and articulate the

MXE experience. Most interesting, using nitrous oxide with MXE will amplify the dissociative, out-of-body effects dramatically, and by breathing in more less of the nitrous oxide one can modulate the experience with a great deal of precision. It can be every bit as transdimensional and otherworldly as DMT or salvia, only the experience is far more euphoric and blissful. I suspect that John Lilly would have loved it.

I've also found that smoking salvia while under the influence of MXE and nitrous oxide works extraordinarily well. The salvia experience is often frightening and not terribly pleasant. The MXE and the nitrous oxide completely eliminate the fear and agitation I often feel after smoking salvia and allow me to observe the extraordinary visions with a sense of emotionally detached curiosity.

I smoked some salvia once after doing MXE and inhaling nitrous oxide and was struck by the profound realization that all I really am, ultimately, is a single cell in the arm of a giant being, who was, at the time, arm wrestling another giant being. My identity fused with the giant being's arm, and it felt so obvious that this was an ultimate truth. It seemed like the mystical oneness that I would normally experience on nitrous oxide, only taken to an even deeper level of reality that I hadn't suspected existed. It became obvious that all of the stress in my life had always resulted from being a tiny part of this tensed-up arm wrestling another arm.

The synergistic MXE–salvia–nitrous oxide experience began like one of my usual nitrous oxide journeys, with a rapid euphoric escalation of realizations and greater and greater insights into the nature of reality, which I only seem to remember when I'm entering nitrous oxide space. This came to its usual mystical climax, where I realized in ecstasy that I was ultimately a part of the one universal consciousness that permeates all of the cosmos and that there is a clever joke hidden in all of this. And then suddenly I realized that everything I thought was contained in that universal consciousness— all that could ever or will ever exist—was itself just embedded within something even larger that I never realized before. That something else was this giant arm involved in an arm-wrestling match. It was extremely weird, and afterward it seemed as if a trickster spirit had been toying with me.

Some of the other combinations that have worked especially well for me are LSD and MDMA (with the MDMA taken around five hours after the LSD), LSD and DMT (with the DMT smoked after the peak of the LSD trip), MDMA and ketamine or MXE (which is a lot like MDMA and nitrous oxide), and LSD and *Salvia divinorum*. I find that LSD works synergistically best with other psychedelics after the acid has peaked. And, of course, cannabis goes well with every psychedelic I've ever tried, helping to heighten, soften, modulate, and integrate the experience.

I've found that the sexually enhancing herb yohimbe goes great with LSD if you'd like to focus a lot of the psychedelic energy through sexual channels, but it should never be mixed with harmaline, MDMA, ketamine, DXM, or MXE. For me the herbs kava, valerian, skullcap, and holy basil can significantly reduce anxiety if a psychedelic experience becomes agitating or difficult, almost as well as Valium. The amino acids L-tryptophan and L-theanine can also be quite helpful in reducing psychedelic anxiety. Several hundred milligrams of niacin (vitamin B₃) will reliably terminate an LSD trip in about thirty minutes for most people, and in cases of severe psychedelic anxiety Valium, Ativan, and GHB appear to work best, if all else fails.

To learn how to deal with a psychedelic emergency I recommend watching the educational film that MAPS made on this subject, titled "Psychedelic Crisis," which can be viewed on YouTube.*

Kratom tea and opium poppy tea are two more of my favorite additions to psychedelic journeys, especially at the end when I'm coming down. High doses of kratom or poppy tea can often induce a lucid

*See www.youtube.com/watch?v=1aBjoARwlOY.

dream–like state that is extremely pleasant, especially when combined with nitrous oxide. Herbs that have subtle psychoactive effects on me normally can have dramatic effects when combined with a psychedelic that amplifies one's sensitivity. This is a topic that should be explored in a whole book.

NUTRITIONAL SUPPORT WITH PSYCHEDELICS

Taking MDMA can be riskier than the classical psychedelics. It's far more toxic, and there is some controversy about it possibly causing lasting brain damage. Unlike marijuana, LSD, and psilocybin, just several times the effective dose of MDMA can be deadly. There's also some concern that when MDMA is absorbed into nerve terminals it causes lasting damage to the dendrites, or connecting fibers with other brain cells, particularly serotonergic dendrites, which release the calming neurotransmitter serotonin.

Research by pharmacologist David E. Nichols at Purdue University demonstrated that taking a single dose of the SSRI antidepressant drug Prozac at the right time can completely prevent this neural damage. The Prozac needs to be taken within six hours of the initial dose of MDMA for this to be effective.

Here's why: MDMA binds to serotonin receptors in the brain, and this causes a part of the brain cells, the serotonin transporters, to work in reverse. That is, for around five or six hours, instead of pumping serotonin back into the nerve terminal as they normally do, the serotonin transporters start pumping serotonin out of the neurons, into the synapse, where it stimulates neighboring cells and produces the desired psychoactive effects. After around six hours the serotonin transporters begin pumping serotonin back into the nerve terminals again, and the MDMA is carried along with the neurotransmitters into the nerve terminal, where it may cause lasting damage. Prozac binds to the same receptor sites in the brain as MDMA, only much more aggressively, and it knocks the MDMA molecules off the receptors before they can be absorbed, so they are safely removed from the body before causing any damage.

Additional studies have shown that large doses of vitamin C and alpha lipoic acid can also prevent any observable damage to serotonergic dendrites from the drug. MDMA is also thought to deplete the body of the important minerals calcium and magnesium, which promotes the commonly experienced jaw clenching, and, of course, it also depletes the body of serotonin, so tryptophan or 5-HTP supplements are also recommended at the end of the experience.

Nitrous oxide use depletes the body of vitamin B_{12}, so if one is doing large amounts of this giggly gas, it would probably be wise to take a sublingual vitamin B_{12} supplement while inhaling the gas.

In general, the healthier your body and mind, the more you will benefit from a psychedelic experience. A large part of my writing career and two of my previous books have been dedicated to health science, alternative medicine, medical breakthroughs, and increasing longevity. I find that maintaining optimal health is an absolute necessity if one is going to continually embark on psychedelic journeys throughout life.

As long as I maintain proper nutritional support and deep spiritual respect, these polypsychedelic combinations have been unusually effective, more than astonishing, and have had lasting benefits. It's where many of the ideas for my science-fiction writings came from. However, there are now many hundreds, or perhaps thousands, of psychonauts on the planet who are far more sophisticated than I in these experiments, as any trip to Erowid will confirm.

The many new designer psychedelics now available appear to show great promise. Some of the more recent psychedelic combinations I've experimented with were designer psychedelics that friends turned me on to. I've particularly enjoyed a tryptamine analog known as 4-HO-MET, which felt like a pleasant mix of MDMA and psilocybin.

RESEARCH CHEMICALS FOR PSYCHONAUTS

THE GLOBAL EXPLOSION OF DESIGNER PSYCHEDELICS
AND SELF-EXPERIMENTATION

Legal and semilegal chemical analogs of psychedelic drugs are readily available on the Internet, and an active online community is experimenting with them and sharing reports. Thanks to extraordinary experimental chemists like *PiHKAL* coauthor Alexander "Sasha" Shulgin and Purdue pharmacologist David E. Nichols, hundreds of new analogs of psilocybin, DMT, LSD, THC, and MDMA have been developed, with a whole range of fascinating effects that deserve further study. Many of these novel drugs are readily available over the Internet from chemical-supply houses, where they are legally sold as research materials and, of course, not for human consumption.

Although most of these drugs have hardly been studied at all, many of them are closely related to chemical compounds known to be fairly safe. However, no one really knows what dangers, health risks, or benefits they may carry.

The new designer psychedelics have names like 4-Acetoxy-DMT, 4-HO-MET, 2C-I, and TMA-2. Sasha's books *PiHKAL* and *TiHKAL,* which he wrote with his wife, Ann, are treasure-filled encyclopedias of reports on hundreds of these compounds, largely derived from two primary classes of chemicals called tryptamines and phenethylamines. (On page 29 of *TiHKAL,* in the section about the DEA raid on the Shulgins' lab—fictionalized, of course—the "Flying High" interview that a DEA agent pulled out of his briefcase was a reference to the 1994 interview Rebecca Novick and I did with the Shulgins that appeared in *High Times* magazine.)

When I interviewed Sasha, I asked him what type of drugs he thought would be developed in the future and if he saw potential for pharmacological tools to be used to expand creativity, intelligence, and spiritual understanding. He said:

I think anything that the human is capable of doing through the mind is duplicable pharmacologically—it's all chemistry upstairs. I think anything from insight to paranoia to joy to fear can all be reproduced chemically. The fact that there are specific receptor sites for specific materials in the body, which duplicate the actions of drugs from outside the body, implies that those receptor sites at which these drugs operate are there because the human produces one for that same purpose.

The Shulgins' books *PiHKAL* and *TiHKAL* also include the chemical instructions for how to synthesize all the pharmacological wonders he designed. On websites like Erowid and Bluelight, a sophisticated community of people using these substances—self-described as psychonauts—discuss their reactions, experiments, mistakes, dosages, and success stories in great detail.

I tried the designer psychedelic 4-HO-MET with great success at the 12 milligram dosage, which is fairly low. As I mentioned earlier, it felt like a wonderful mixture of psilocybin and MDMA to me and greatly facilitated social bonding and emotional intimacy with a close friend. Another designer psychedelic that I tried and really enjoyed goes by the name Foxy, and it's a tryptamine chemically called 5-MeO-DIPT, which felt like a similar but different blend of MDMA-like and psychedelic effects, only with a distinctive skin-sensitizing, erotically arousing dimension. It seems like there are endless variations and combinations of what's possible by chemically reconfiguring our brains.

A 2011 article on WebMD, "New Black Market Designer Drugs: Why Now?" warned against the potential health dangers of these new designer psychedelics as well as their potential political threat to FDA-approved, medical psychedelic drug research. Prominent psychedelic drug researchers quoted in the article agreed that the wide use of these newly crafted molecules could damage the warming political climate toward the medical use of psychedelics.

After an eighteen-year worldwide ban on clinical psychedelic drug research, there is now a scientific renaissance occurring—with LSD, MDMA, and psilocybin studies—and some people are concerned that this rise in nonclinical, unauthorized psychedelic experimentation could shift the political climate away from approving the studies and reinforcing the ban.

The author of the WebMD article, Daniel J. DeNoon, stated, "Society's reaction to rampant illicit use of psychedelic drugs derailed research from the early 1970s until the mid-1990s. It remains to be seen whether the current surge in illicit designer drugs once again creates a backlash that makes legitimate research impossible." (Actually, human psychedelic research began again in 1990 with Rick Strassman's DMT study at the University of New Mexico.)

While I certainly won't downplay the potential dangers of taking an unstudied drug or in any way condone any illegal activity, and I understand very well that clinical psychedelic research was banned for many years as a political backlash against their use by the counterculture, I couldn't disagree with DeNoon more. Arguably most sports are more physically dangerous than psychedelic drugs, and there are more hospital visits every year from high school cheerleading injuries than from dangerous reactions to psychedelic drugs.

As readers of this book are becoming increasingly aware, I strongly suspect that psychedelic drugs are catalyzing the evolution of consciousness on this planet in a profound, dramatic, necessary, and extremely positive way. It's simply a force of nature that governments are powerless to stop, and I certainly wouldn't rely on FDA-approved, corporation-funded, academic scientists to lead the way.

I think that psychedelic drugs and plants are our best hope for raising ecological awareness, for dissolving the cultural boundaries that separate us, for enhancing our creative potential and spiritually realigning our largely parasitic species with the rest of the biosphere, before it's too late.

I think the brave individuals who have courageously experimented with these novel psychedelic drugs should be considered heroic explorers, like Sir Francis Drake or Ferdinand Magellan, charting the unknown topography of these new states of consciousness and helping us to establish a symbiotic relationship with the rest of the biosphere. People seem to forget that all of the medical studies with psychedelics that are currently going on largely resulted from reports that came from brave explorers who engaged in illegal, forbidden, and unauthorized forms of self-exploration with these remarkable substances.

I don't think that there would even be any scientific studies going on today had it not been for all the people who used it illegally, in nonclinical settings, and reported positive benefits that they thought could help others. How else would we even know that LSD can help with cluster headaches or MDMA with PTSD?

Also, it's not unusual for some chemists to experiment on themselves; there is a long historical tradition of this. Albert Hofmann, the Swiss chemist who discovered LSD, tried it on himself first. All of the different phenethylamines and tryptamines that are discussed in Shulgin's books were first personally tested by him and a small research group of his friends. The first psychedelic plants were likely discovered by accidental ingestion before we were even human, and this led to deliberate ingestions long before any scientific studies.

Sure, doing unstudied psychedelic drugs—especially in the wrong dosages or in improper settings—can be risky and dangerous; no one will argue with that. But not doing psychedelic drugs can also be dangerous. Psychedelics tend to dissolve the mental boundaries of ecological blindness, psychological imprints, and cultural conditioning that cause us to feel, think, and act mechanically in unhealthy ways.

I think people who haven't had a psychedelic experience tend to be more vulnerable to rigid, dogmatic ways of thinking, and psychedelics, by their very nature, cause people to question cultural values. Governments and organized religious institutions are acutely aware of this, as I discussed earlier, and I think that's primarily why they're illegal.

The unhealthy psychological and cultural belief systems that we learn as children, without our consent, are contributing to the destruction of our global biosphere, which sustains us and all life on the planet. Psychedelics give us a valuable opportunity to temporarily transcend our selfish, individual viewpoints, see the bigger picture, and recognize our true interconnection with the holy web of life.

Most of my psychedelic journeys have been conducted alone, although more than a few of my combined and synergistic experiences with psychedelics were done with lovers, and sex and psychedelics is another subject that has long fascinated me.

7
Exploring the Synergistic World of Sex on Drugs

Few things in life feel better than getting high and getting laid. My dear friend and renowned sex expert Annie Sprinkle has quoted me on this statement a number of times as we both agree on this and that combining these two ancient forms of pleasures can lead to ecstatic experiences that defy description and bring users closer to the divine.

Annie, whom I first met at a tantric wedding in Maui for our mutual friends Kutira Decosterd and Raphael, is one of the world's experts on human sexuality; a brilliantly creative, ecologically aware artist and activist; and one of the most golden-hearted people that I know.

Annie began her career as a popular porn star, where she received enormous acclaim and celebrity status. In midcareer, due to the medical crisis of a loved one, Annie completely transformed and redesigned herself, metamorphosing from a porn star into a celebrated spiritual-sex teacher and performance artist. I have enormous admiration, respect, and appreciation for Annie's wonderful work and consider her a dear friend. Early in my career as a struggling writer she sent me money to help with my rent when I was too broke to afford it, and she patiently sat on the phone with me one night for hours when I was completely drunk, sobbing to her over a girl who had just left me. I consider Annie to be a true bodhisattva, an enlightened being who returns to this earthly realm to help all sentient beings attain Buddhahood.

I first interviewed Annie for my second interview book, *Voices from the Edge*. After she spoke about her experiences trying psychedelics when she was younger, I asked her about what type of relationship she saw between sex and psychedelics. She replied, "Yeah, there is some connection. When I'm in a state of sexual ecstasy and I get up and look at the moon, I have a psychedelic experience of the moon." This was a fairly tame response, and since then she has become more outspoken about the potentials and pitfalls of combining psychedelics and sex, even writing an article about her experiences with sex and psychedelics for the *MAPS Bulletin*.

Annie and I also taught several well-attended workshops together in San Francisco about what happens when people combine sex and drugs, and a large portion of these sessions focused on what happens when people combine sex and psychedelics. There were some very lively discussions. I learned that for every drug that exists—including cough medicine, antidepressants, and antibiotics—there's someone out there who thinks it's an aphrodisiac. A website was built from the information that we presented at these workshops—www.sex anddrugs.info—and someday we plan to coauthor a book together on this subject.

Psychedelics can enhance every aspect of the sexual experience—physically, emotionally, psychologically, and spiritually. Cannabis and LSD are especially known, legendary some would say, for enhancing sexual sensations, and, in my experience, adding the African herb yohimbe to the mix can certainly heighten the experiences dramatically. I have had more than a dozen utterly amazing orgasms in a single night with LSD. The erotic sequences in my science-fiction novels *Brainchild* and *Virus: The Alien Strain* were based on somewhat exaggerated personal experiences I had while tripping with my lovers. The possibilities that emerge when combining sex with psychedelics clearly defy description, because such powerful and profound forms of ecstasy and unity become so astonishing and all encompassing, though I've tried my best to find words to artistically describe these amazing experiences in my novels.

FORBIDDEN KNOWLEDGE AND ANCIENT SECRETS

Naturally my experiences with sex and psychedelics got me interested in tantra, the ancient Indian system of sexual yoga. Over the years I have become fairly well-acquainted with basic tantric practices and have gotten to know a number of prominent people in the tantric community. This sensual and spiritual community incorporates consciousness-raising sexuality into their daily religious practice. From spending time with these gentle people and being privileged to be allowed to participate in some of their beautiful ceremonies, I learned that it is not uncommon for practitioners of tantra to incorporate psychedelic plants such as cannabis or psilocybin mushrooms into their sacred rituals.

Although the ritualistic mixing of sex and psychedelics is ancient—and openly discussed in the writings of iconoclastic philosophers like Aleister Crowley and my late friend Robert Anton Wilson—the psychopharmacological techniques for activating these higher states of consciousness remain unknown by most people, and they are often kept secret from early initiates of tantra. Techniques for enhancing sexual rituals with sacred plants are rarely mentioned in popular books on tantra or in tantra workshops, and if they are, they are usually discouraged.

This important omission or discouragement is deliberate, although it's sometimes said with a wink to those who are in the know. This is because a good bit of training and mental preparation are required to handle the enormous amount of energy that a tantric-psychedelic session can generate. Tantric sex can be quite intense on its own, and that may be more than enough for most people who are interested in exploring tantra. Not everyone can handle shivering in ecstasy for hours while their partner's face is melting.

The omission of psychedelics is also largely due to the fact that most people in the tantric community are acutely aware that the idea of a sexually based spirituality is controversial enough for most people; mixing sex and religion elicits strong cultural taboos in many people. Making it widely known that some of those same people who are mixing sex and religion are also using Schedule I drugs may not be the wisest way to gain social acceptance during a time in history when sacred plants are regarded as forbidden fruit by the puritanical overlords of society. So their secrecy is understandable.

However, because it can be emotionally risky to mix sex and psychedelics if one isn't properly prepared, perhaps a more open discussion of these experiences would be beneficial, which is why I write so openly about all this, as Robert Anton Wilson did. Because nothing is going to stop people from mixing sex with just about every substance imaginable, and because the emotional consequences of these experiences can be so extreme, openly sharing our experiences with one another is probably a good idea.

PSYCHEDELICS AND MASTURBATION

Here's a subject that I've never seen discussed before: using psychedelics to enhance masturbatory self-pleasure. When I've tripped alone masturbation always played a vital role. It releases deeply clogged kundalini energies and can be enormously pleasurable. It also enhances the power of my imagination and helps me to balance the intense psychedelic energies, which can sometimes become too agitating. I'm aware that a number of other people have discovered this as well.

Pornography comes to life on LSD—fully three-dimensional, animated, almost personally intimate, and one's heightened fantasies blend seamlessly with reality. It's easy to glimpse where future technologies might be headed with the fruitful development of virtual reality, advanced robotics, and even better psychedelics.

Of course, nothing can possibly substitute for the soul-to-soul connection that occurs when two transcendental spirits sexually merge on psychedelics and unify to the core of their beings. A sexual orgasm is naturally psychedelic in the sense that it allows us to temporarily transcend our ego-based consciousness, blend personal boundaries, and merge our consciousness with another. It also allows us to experience a kind of death and rebirth, after which lovers tend to imprint one another sexually, like young children.

It's always been especially interesting to me that the French refer to an orgasm as *la petite mort,* or "the little death."

SEX, DEATH, AND EVOLUTION

When I interviewed artist and tantra expert Penny Slinger, she told me:

> People often talk of sex being like a little death, but seeing as I don't remember my last death at this point, I can't really say for sure. It is said that the initiation your mother gives you through her yoni is one that confers forgetfulness of your past deaths, and this opens the world for you for your new incarnation. So I don't know if the experience is exactly similar. Other people have also said that psychedelics are again like a little death. So sex and drugs may have some connection to death, in the sense that they can create a portal into the world which is full of energy and magic, the intangible and the unknown. The biggest taboos in our society are around these things because people tend to fear the unknown.

The synergistic combinations of sex and drugs that have intrigued me for so long have led me to speculate on the fact that sex and death are so deeply linked in our evolutionary past and are so intimately connected in our culture, because they arrived together simultaneously in our evolution.

202 ● Exploring the Synergistic World of Sex on Drugs

Aside from what occurred from reckless behavior, before sexual reproduction, all living organisms were basically immortal. Asexual organisms just grow until they divide. They grow and split, grow and split, forever and ever—or until they're eaten by other organisms or are accidentally killed. The price of sexual reproduction is that each individual organism must get old and die.

From the point of view of individual consciousness, aging and death may seem like a pretty steep price to pay for the ability to orgasm and swap genes, although it's also inspiring to realize that all living beings are born out of a moment of passion and ecstasy, that each human life is created through the magic of orgasms and love. Orgasms create organisms. All of us are the result of countless beings loving one another.

It could be that sexuality, aging, and death mark the beginning of another evolutionary process that our limited monkey minds have yet to understand. Regardless, I think that the simultaneous appearance of sex and death in our evolutionarily past is what makes it remain so intimately linked in our culture, although, as with many obvious observations that threaten our fragile realities, we generally don't recognize this.

So many cultural references to sexuality continuously zip around our conscious awareness and influence us subconsciously, and many advertisers are eager to exploit our sexual vulnerabilities to market their products. One particularly striking example of a blatant cultural reference to sexuality that often goes unnoticed as such is the Valentine's Day heart, which bears no physical resemblance whatsoever to the cardiac organ that beats in our chest and circulates our blood. Where did this ever-so-popular and beloved image come from? We see it everywhere. Timothy Leary pointed out to me that what this ancient symbol really appears to be is a fully extended female sex organ, an erotically excited vulva engorged with red blood, being pierced with a magical phallic arrow of love.

If we take an evolutionary view sexuality, like intelligence, appears to be increasing across species over time, and if we continue with our teleological perspective, it seems that genetic intelligence has something in mind here. Humans are one of the few species that are in heat, so to speak, all year round and are always sexually active, always ready to engage in erotic exchanges, and forever fantasizing about them. We often take this erotic eagerness for granted, but most animals just go into heat for a few months or weeks a year.

If you look at the evolution of animal bodies, two characteristics that have increased over the eons are the physical size of the brain and of our sexual organs. You can actually chart them right next to each other and see their mutual rise relative to other organs in the body. It seems like this is something that DNA or genetic intelligence had in mind, and we can only speculate where it's going.

Throughout evolution there has also been a greater frequency of sexual activity as well as a greater duration of time in which the animals are in heat—peaking with animals who are in heat basically all the time. Now human beings are devoting even more time and energy to sexual activity, and we appear to be trying to increase these desires and abilities even more by developing new drugs and new technologies that increase our potency and enhance our experience.

A whole new homegrown science has been enthusiastically built around what are called *prosexual drugs,* a term coined by my friend John Morgenthaler, who also coined the term *smart drugs* for drugs that improve cognitive function and overall brain performance. Many of the same drugs that improve cognitive abilities, interestingly enough, also improve sexual performance.

Combining some of these drugs with psychedelics, especially LSD, can provide for extraordinary experiences, as many can attest. One drug in particular, cabergoline, allows men to have multiple orgasms like women, because it blocks the release of the orgasm-inhibiting hormone prolactin. This subject has been explored in depth in John Morgenthaler and Dan Joy's marvelous book *Better Sex through Chemistry* (which I highly recommend, although it is a bit outdated), and my articles on the subject can be easily found online. Low doses of ibogaine, a powerful psychedelic derived from the African iboga plant, is also known to be a powerful sexual stimulant.

But back to the intimately intertwined subjects of sex and death. I think that a sizable number of people often confuse this ancient evolutionary connection with sex and violence, but this cultural connection—largely associated with sex crimes and often linked in film, television, and other popular forms of media—is, I think, the result of very different causes. I suspect that there is actually an inverse relationship between sex and violence. In other words, cultures that are more open sexually, where sexuality is less inhibited and more freely engaged in, experience less violence. Further, I suspect that most of the violence in the world is caused by sexually frustrated teenage boys. Crime statistics show that most violent crimes are caused by teenage boys or men in their early twenties, when sexual desire is generally at its peak. Cultures that embrace a more open attitude toward sexuality appear to experience significantly less violence than cultures that have strong taboos and prohibitions against it.

WHERE WERE THE BONOBOS IN
THE PLANET OF THE APES?

I think that we're currently living on the Planet of the Apes, because I feel like I'm genetically wired and have been subculturally reinforced to see the present state of our world as barbaric and primitive, like I'm the Great Gazoo living in a *Flintstones* cartoon. Every time I see the film footage of those menacing gorilla soldiers in the classic film *Planet of the Apes* (which I absolutely loved as a child), using wooden clubs to bash the poor, innocent, peaceful, war-protesting chimpanzees and brutally slaughtering humans as game animals, I always envision DEA (Drug Enforcement Agency) insignias on their black leather military jackets. However, in reality, chimps are not exactly the most peaceful of primate species.

The differences between the two similar primate species—chimpanzees and bonobos—provide enormous insight into human behavior, because these are the two species that are most closely related to us evolutionarily and genetically. And, fascinatingly, they take virtually 180-degree approaches to sexuality and its role in their communal societies, which has a dramatic effect on how the two different animals cooperate with one another. Their approaches are almost embarrassingly mirrored among human societies. The two types of societies that author Riane Eisler describes as partnership and dominator in her book *The Chalice and the Blade* seem to reflect a similar pattern among primates.

In dominator societies men rule over women and other men, and some men have enormous power and control over others. In partnership societies there is mutual cooperation between both sexes and all people have equal rights. According to Eisler, whom I interviewed for my book *Mavericks of the Mind,* most societies in the world today are dominator societies, but in the past partnership societies—such as in Minoan Crete—have flourished.

Terence McKenna believed that the shift away from using boundary-dissolving shamanic plants, such as cannabis and magic mushrooms, and the move toward using alcohol as society's primary recreational drug of choice is what largely caused the change from partnership to dominator societies. At modern psychedelic festivals like Burning Man, Earthdance, and the Rainbow Gatherings, it seems like a partnership model of society can indeed work and that liberated sexuality and psychedelic drugs really do seem to foster a more cooperative society.

The famous 1969 music festival in Woodstock, New York, and the 1968 Summer of Love in San Francisco's Golden Gate Park were the beginning of a resurgence in partnership societies, an archaic revival, as McKenna called it, that is flourishing today. These peaceful, cooperative festivals, where a large percentage of the participants are tripping on psychedelics, have been happening all over the globe for the past forty-five years. They occur in makeshift tribal communities that are commonly referred to as "temporary autonomous zones," a term coined by writer Hakim Bey that describes what many raves, alternative-culture festivals, rock concerts, and other radical experiments in social freedom have in common.

Chimpanzee societies are ruled by an alpha male and they are a lot like dominator societies, whereas bonobos are socially egalitarian and partnership oriented. Females rule in bonobo societies, and sexual pleasure is used among its groups as a way to resolve important conflicts. In addition to reproduction and conflict resolution, it also appears that bonobos engage in sexual activities simply for pleasure and pure enjoyment. Chimps frequently engage in violence among one another, and there are often murders and even wars between them. Bonobos, on the other hand, are rarely violent toward one another, and instead they frequently engage in sexual behaviors together, on average around every three hours.

If two groups of chimps meet for the first time a ferocious battle is likely to ensue. However, when two bonobo groups first encounter one another it's more likely that a wild orgy will break out.

All kinds of sexual behaviors occur between bonobos, such as face-to-face sex, group sex, bisexuality, oral sex, and masturbation with toys—many of the behaviors that a lot of people thought were unique to human beings and many that are clearly not for reproductive purposes. Every member of a bonobo group has sex with every other member, regardless of gender or age, and this helps to facilitate social bonding. Bonobos appear to have found a way to resolve interpersonal conflicts without resorting to violence, as chimps do, and these hippielike animals are truly the "make love, not war" species of primates. I think we can learn a lot from them.

A comparative analysis of bonobo and chimpanzee brains shows anatomical differences that may be responsible for their differing social behaviors. According to Emory University anthropologist James Rilling, who led the analysis, "The neural circuitry that mediates anxiety, empathy, and the inhibition of aggression in humans is better developed in bonobos than in chimpanzees."*

If bonobos, rather than chimps, gorillas, and orangutans, were the primate ancestors that spawned the rulers in *Planet of the Apes,* the world that evolved may have been much more peaceful and fun. Something to think about when we reflect on the differences between political attitudes among human beings and where our own future evolution may be headed.

PLANET EARTH'S FIRST TRULY PSYCHEDELIC CIVILIZATION: BLACK ROCK CITY

In 2008 I went to the Burning Man Festival in the Black Rock Desert of Nevada for the first time, and this turned out to be one of the most incredible experiences of my life. I stayed in Entheon Village, where MAPS was based and where one of the largest theme camps in Black Rock City is located each year. I spent a lot of time just exploring the ephemeral city and taking it all in. The environment there was certainly a huge challenge for me, but it was also unusually rewarding—truly spectacular in so many ways—and I had a profound experience there that deeply renewed my sense of hope in the future evolution of the human species.

The Black Rock Desert is a flat, 400-square-mile, prehistoric lake bed that's completely devoid of any vegetation or animal habitats, and the weather conditions there were pretty much the worst that I've ever experienced. It felt like landing on Mars or in the postapocalyptic, globally warmed remains of a dead biosphere. On my first day there a wild and windy six-hour dust storm hit. It was well over 100 degrees, and the alkaline dust was so thick in the air that I could barely see more than a few feet in front of me. The playa dust gets into and permeates everything, making it impossible to stay clean. It was not a terribly pleasant

*See "Clues to Human Social Brain Found in Chimps and Bonobos," http://ts-si .org/neuroscience/29567-clues-to-human-social-brain-found-in-chimps-and-bonobos (accessed January 7, 2013).

experience, lying in a domed tent or wandering about outside, wearing a pair of ski goggles and a wet bandana over my nose, in the midst of this blinding chaos.

Then when the sun went down the temperature dropped to around 40 degrees but felt much colder when the strong, dry winds blew across the playa. In addition to these less-than-ideal weather conditions, the whole week was an intensely socially overloading, noisy, sleep-depriving experience. Burning Man is no pleasure cruise, that's for sure. At the same time, being in Entheon Village with my good friends from MAPS, I couldn't possibly have been staying with better camp mates or have had better resources available to me.

Despite all these challenges Burning Man was also beautiful and enriching! Simply spending a week in Black Rock City can be as profoundly transformative as a psychedelic experience. Like an LSD journey, it's difficult to describe this enchanted place in words. Burning Man really has to be experienced to be understood. It's a magical place where synchronicities and surprises abound. I went there primarily to see the artwork—which is truly beyond spectacular, absolutely incredible. Photographs simply can't capture the immensity and the wonderfully animated, unearthly insanity of it all. It's the collective imagination materialized, where every cultural icon from your childhood, every strange interdimensional archetype, and every beyond-belief psychedelic vision is brought to life in a deliciously surreal circus. Hands down, it's the greatest art show on Earth; the Louvre doesn't even compare.

But what struck me most about Burning Man, what really inspired me, was the incredible sense of community, the enormous amount of generosity, and the fact that at least for one week a year a truly psychedelic civilization is possible on planet Earth.

Black Rock City is the planet's first truly psychedelic civilization. The psychedelic imagination becomes tangible there, no money exchange or bartering is allowed, and there is a feeling of almost complete freedom. Everyone there simply shares their gifts, their visions, and their creativity with everyone else—similar to how the DMT elves in hyperspace have often been described—and it works! Almost everyone there is psychedelically experienced and unusually creative. It's a whole city, almost fifty thousand people, of psychedelic artists. A post-terrestrial, post-survival society built upon the spirit of a simple aspiration: to delight and marvel the senses, to blow people's minds.

It feels as though a powerful morphic field is created in Black Rock City; gathering so many electrified nervous systems in one place seems to accelerate and elevate everyone's consciousness. All the people I spoke with reported feeling high, whether or not they did psychedelics. And I now realize that the very things that prevented me from going all these years—the expense, all the necessary preparations and time off from work, the extremely harsh environmental conditions—are actually deterrents that weed out anyone who doesn't really want to be there. So the people who make it there are generally pretty special. Evolutionarily speaking, the citizens of Black Rock City are akin to the first fish that crawled out of the sea on to dry land. Burning Man's geographic destiny lies in high orbit, in the heavens, among the stars.

Attending Burning Man was spiritually transformative. I suspect that the playa dust in the Black Rock desert may also be psychoactive, as the whole experience feels like a psychedelic trip. I met so many extraordinary people from all over the world, made strong new connections, and had a powerful mystical experience while watching the Temple burn on the final night.

It didn't occur to me until I was tripping at the festival (on a popular MDMA analog called 2C-B) and watching the giant straw man burn that the Man largely represents the establishment culture. When the Man burns on Saturday night, it's the wildest party on Earth, but when the Temple burns on the following night, and burners ritualistically release their grief into the fire, almost everyone there is totally silent. It was truly a shamanic journey, and I felt an overwhelming sense of love for everyone there. When I got back home I wasn't able to tell people about my experience at Burning Man for the first few days without crying, I was so deeply moved by it all. In retrospect it's hard to believe that it really happened, because the experience had such a dreamlike quality to it.

Black Rock City explores the radical potentials of human culture and the possibilities for our future evolution when our species' imagination becomes physically tangible. However, thinking back to our earlier evolutionary origins helps to elevate another universal dream to the surface of our collective awareness as a realistic possibility: the desire for immortality. With the exception of a planetary holocaust, DNA is already immortal, and before sexual reproduction evolved, so, potentially, were all living creatures.

Timothy Leary summarized what he thought the teleological goals of DNA and the evolutionary process were in the clever acronym SMI^{2}LE. This stood for *space migration, intelligence increase* (or *intelligence squared*), and *life extension*. We've discussed space migration as part of DNA's goal to "get high," and immortality is clearly something that the human spirit also deeply craves—and ultimately strives for in the earthly realm, as is evidenced by the role of our culture's most revered institution: medicine.

REACHING TOWARD IMMORTALITY

Tell me: What is the number-one killer of human beings in the world?

If you answered heart disease, cancer, AIDS, accidents, environmental toxins, or wars, you missed the obvious. Hands down, the number-one human killer is, of course, the aging process. Aging makes us more vulnerable to diseases and accidents. Slowing down or reversing the aging process would be the most naturally effective approach to curing almost all diseases, and this valuable insight has been an important theme in much of my work. It was the subject of two of my past books, *Mavericks of Medicine* and *Detox through Oral Chelation*.

I've also written many dozens of articles about the benefits of cognitive enhancers like Hydergine, Deprenyl, and Piracetam (my three personal favorites); the intelligent use of nutritional supplements, medicinal herbs, and little-known forms of alternative medicine; as well as the new, cutting-edge technologies that are creating medical break-throughs. I suspect that within the next few decades, if not sooner, all human diseases will become curable, and the aging process itself will become reversible.

Like technology expert Ray Kurzweil, whom I interviewed for two of my books, I believe that physical immortality will be developed in successively more successful stages and that staying alive as long as possible will give us the greatest opportunity to be around when the most important breakthroughs in nanotechnology and genetic engineering come along.

Perhaps the most compelling reason why radical life extension appears possible for us is because not all animals age like we do. In fact it seems that some animals don't age at all. When I interviewed John Guerin, director of the Ageless Animals Project, he told me about rockfish caught off the coast of Alaska that were hundreds of years old, healthy, and fertile. Whales have been known to live for more than two hundred years without showing any signs of aging. A male whale that was more than a hundred years old was harpooned while it was in the midst of having sex. Guerin believes that by study-ing these types of animals we can learn why they live so long without losing vitality or fertility and then apply that knowledge to extending the life span of human beings.

Kurzweil spoke to me about how nanotechnology, artificial intel-ligence, and advanced robotics will eventually allow humans to live for indefinite periods of time without aging. Kurzweil thinks that "nanobots, blood cell–size devices that could go inside the body and keep us healthy from inside," will be available in about two decades. So Kurzweil believes that if we can just stay alive for another fifteen or twenty years we'll be able to live forever.

Nanotechnology would not only allow for radical life extension but also for a dramatic improvement in all physical capabilities, including brain functions. Kurzweil believes that the line between biology and technology is going to completely blur together in the decades to come and that nanotechnological brain implants will substantially increase our intelligence and dramatically expand the power of the human mind. The power of the mind and its relationship to medicine is another important theme in my work, which I discussed at the beginning of this chapter in the section on mind-body medicine.

Perhaps even more fascinating than mind-body medicine is a transpersonal phenomenon known as remote healing. It seems that what we think may not only affect our own health, but it also may directly affect the health of others. When I interviewed Larry Dossey he told me about numerous controlled, double-blind studies demonstrating that prayer can have measurable health effects. The effects of directing positive intention have been demonstrated in dozens of controlled laboratory studies in people, animals, and even bacteria.

Dossey also told me about studies that demonstrated health benefits from engaging in religious practice and spoke about the integration of medicine with spirituality. Reflecting on the integration of medicine with spirituality brings one to the notion that sometimes healing the essence of who we are and reducing suffering, may mean letting go of the physical body.

THE RIGHT TO DIE

Just because medical technologies give us the ability to live forever doesn't mean that we have to do so. Timothy Leary was one of the first people to start promoting ideas about life extension; he began doing so in the late 1970s. He believed attaining physical immortality was one of the "goals" of biological evolution. Leary's enthusiasm inspired longevity researchers and helped to popularize transhumanist ideas about how science would soon conquer the aging process and allow us to virtually live forever.

However, when Leary was diagnosed with terminal prostate cancer at age seventy-six, he said that he was "thrilled and ecstatic" to hear that he was going die. As much as Leary loved life—which I can personally attest to—he not only accepted death but also embraced it. In the end he even decided to forgo his plans for cryonic suspension. I think there is an important lesson in Leary's dying process about the importance of facing the mystery of death with the same openness and sense of adventure with which one faces life.

In other words, attaining physical immortality in a human body may not be the final stage for evolving consciousness in this universe. Numerous spiritual traditions, such as Hinduism and many forms of shamanism, assert that healing the spirit sometimes involves transcending the body and moving on to whatever is after death. However, regardless of whether consciousness survives death, not everyone may wish to hang around until the final collapse of the universe, and certainly people who are in chronic pain or who are suffering greatly should be given the option to leave if they wish.

When I asked Weil about his views on the controversial issue of euthanasia he said:

> I don't think it's appropriate for doctors to be involved in that, although I think patients should be able to discuss that issue with doctors. I think that for people with overwhelming diseases, for whom life has become really difficult, that they should have that choice, and that there should be mechanisms provided for helping them with that.

Jack Kevorkian, on the other hand, believed that physicians should be able to perform euthanasia and was in prison for second-degree murder because he assisted with the last wish of a patient who was suffering from ALS. When I interviewed Kevorkian about voluntary death for my book *Mavericks of Medicine,* I learned that, despite the U.S. government and medical establishment's opposition to euthanasia, 80 percent of the public support a patient's right to die, and one in five physicians has admitted to practicing euthanasia at some point in their career. Why, then, is euthanasia illegal? Kevorkian said:

> I think that the U.S. government, medical establishment, and pharmaceutical companies are opposed to euthanasia for monetary or financial reasons. To help correct this situation there has to be an organized public response and outcry—which I believe is now occurring.

While the goals of contemporary Western medicine are healing disease and treating injuries, the goals that one aspires to in the pursuit of optimal health are much larger and more encompassing. This may involve developing an immortal, nanotechnologically proficient, self-repairing superbody of our own design, or it may involve gracefully transcending this world entirely and discarding our body like a pile of used clothing. But either way I think that the primary goal of medicine should be the reduction of human suffering. I think that if we make the reduction of human suffering our number-one priority, the future of medicine does indeed appear very bright.

THE FUTURE OF MEDICINE

We are living in truly astonishing times. Although our current health care system appears to be crumbling around us, we are simultaneously witnessing a rapidly advancing biotechnology revolution that promises to forever change the course of human history. New possibilities are emerging everywhere we turn, and there is enormous cause for hope. When we look out onto the frontiers of medicine we see an incredible vista blossoming with possibilities that stagger the mind and border on the miraculous. New advances in medicine promise to help humanity end countless generations of suffering and deliver us into a golden age where disease and aging are merely subjects that we learn about in history class, and the boundaries of our physical capacities are limited only by our imaginations.

However, death appears to be an inevitable fact of nature, something that we all ultimately must face, and I think it's something that is best not be feared. So let's open-mindedly explore what may or may not happen to consciousness after physical death, which is the subject of my next chapter.

8

What Happens to Consciousness after Death?

Considering that the dying process is probably the most universally feared of all human experiences, that the death of loved ones causes more suffering in this world than anything else, and that death is an inevitable fact of nature, it seems like it might be a good idea to pay close attention to what researchers have learned about how psychedelics can help ease the dying process.

There is an abundance of scientific and historical evidence and countless anecdotal reports that testify to the fact that cannabis and psychedelics can help ease the suffering of those who are dying. This was the subject of a theme bulletin that I edited for MAPS in 2009, and I wrote a chapter about it for the book *The Natural Death Handbook* in 2012.

Some of the most valuable and promising research that's been conducted with psychedelics has been in the area of treating the terminally ill. For example, the studies conducted with terminally ill patients by psychiatric researcher Stanislav Grof and medical anthropologist Joan Halifax at Spring Grove State Hospital in Baltimore provided strong evidence that a psychedelic experience can be immensely beneficial for people in their final stages of life.

Between the years 1967 and 1972 studies with terminal cancer patients by Grof, Halifax, and colleagues showed that LSD combined with psychotherapy could alleviate symptoms of depression, tension, anxiety, sleep disturbances, psychological withdrawal, and even severe physical pain that was resistant to opiates. If all this wasn't enough to hail the treatment as miraculous, it also significantly improved communication between the patients and their loved ones.

In addition to LSD and other potent psychedelics, the milder and gentler cannabis plant can also provide enormous relief from many illnesses, and it too can often help ease the suffering of those who are dying.

I've written numerous articles about the many medical benefits of cannabis, its remarkable safety, and how totally outrageous the criminal laws against it are. The two main reasons why cannabis is still illegal are that too many influential people are profiting from its illegal status, and there's a legitimate fear (by those in power) that cannabis use causes people to question cultural values. In a healthy culture we would welcome this natural inquiry and use it to continuously redefine ourselves so that we improve and become better and better at what we do. But for people who have a lot invested in the power structure as it currently is, they may see cannabis use as a serious threat to political and corporate value systems.

Nonetheless, at the time of this writing the walls of cannabis prohibition are beginning to seriously crumble, and it isn't likely that they'll continue to stand for very much longer, as every day more and more people are in favor of legalization.

As a proud member of the Wo/Men's Alliance for Medical Marijuana (WAMM) since 1997, I've also personally witnessed how cannabis can help ease the dying process. WAMM is a Santa Cruz–based, medical marijuana collective, and it is the most highly praised, unique, and successful of all medical marijuana organizations in the world. WAMM members receive medicinal cannabis at production cost in exchange for volunteer work. There is no charge for members who are too ill to work, and the organization is not only strongly supported by the community but also by the local government. It is considered an essential component of the Santa Cruz medical system, and I feel honored to be a part of it.

Many of the people in WAMM are dying from terminal illnesses, and one can clearly see how much the cannabis is helping to relieve a lot of their pain and suffering on many levels—physically, emotionally, and spiritually. WAMM's cofounder, Valerie Leveroni Corral, is one of my personal heroines and dearest friends. I've seen Valerie almost every Tuesday evening since 1997 at the weekly WAMM meetings, which always end with the same cheer.

ONE, TWO, THREE—WAMM!

Valerie Leveroni Corral was the first person in California to challenge the marijuana laws in court, based on the necessity defense, common-law doctrine dating to the Magna Carta, and win. She also helped lead the 1996 battle to pass Proposition 215, the state's medical marijuana law. An article in the *New York Times* referred to Corral as "the Florence Nightingale and Johnny Appleseed of medical marijuana rolled into one." And according to *High Times* magazine, "Valerie's leadership role in the battle for medical marijuana is unquestioned."

Valerie was in a serious automobile accident in 1973 that left her so severely epileptic that she often suffered from five grand mal seizures a day. With "deliberate application and mindful monitoring," Valerie began using cannabis as an adjunct medicine to help control her seizures in 1974. This treatment soon replaced her rigorous pharmaceutical regimen, and it eventually became the sole medication that she has used to control her seizures for more than a decade.

Valerie and her husband, Mike, were arrested in 1992 for the cultivation of five marijuana plants. As a result of this arrest and her historical victory in in court, Valerie was ushered into the legal, political, and social spotlight of the medical marijuana health issue.

Valerie was helpful in changing the law of California with Proposition 215, which allows people with serious illnesses to use marijuana with the recommendation of a physician. Understanding that a lack of financial resources prevented many needy and deserving patients from receiving high-priced medical marijuana, Valerie was instrumental in drafting the provision in Proposition 215 that allows patients and their caregivers to cultivate their own medicine.

WAMM was founded in 1993 in Santa Cruz. Later that year Valerie and Mike were again arrested for cultivation and distribution to other patients. But no jury in California would ever convict the Corrals, the DA dropped the case, and WAMM flourished. WAMM differs from other medical marijuana organizations in that it is entirely patient and caregiver run. The majority of patients in WAMM suffer from cancer or AIDS, although a number of the members suffer from other serious ailments such as epilepsy, glaucoma, and multiple sclerosis. The organization provides marijuana at no cost to more than two hundred patients, who share in the cultivation, distribution, and fund-raising that keeps the organization alive. WAMM is also generously supported by the local community and law enforcement of Santa Cruz.

On September 5, 2002, federal agents from the DEA raided the WAMM garden and the Corral's home with automatic weapons and full-on riot gear. They seized all of the plants, leaving nearly 250 seriously ill people without medicine, and took Valerie and Mike away in handcuffs. In an unprecedented show of community support, forty WAMM members blocked the DEA in the WAMM garden with their bodies and wheelchairs across the only road off the property and refused to leave until Valerie and Mike were released. The couple was released that afternoon, and a flurry of media activity followed.

In response to their arrest the city of Santa Cruz allowed WAMM to distribute marijuana on the steps of city hall on September 17. WAMM became engaged in a lawsuit against the federal government for their right to use medical marijuana, and the City Council of Santa Cruz, as well as the County of Santa Cruz, signed on to this historic lawsuit acknowledging WAMM as an integral part of the Santa Cruz health care system. In this high-profile case, *County of Santa Cruz et al. v. Ashcroft,* Judge Jeremy Fogel of the Northern District of California granted the plaintiffs a preliminary injunction and denied the government's motion to dismiss the plaintiffs' complaint. Although WAMM eventually lost the case at the level of the Supreme Court, this temporary ruling protected WAMM while the lawsuit was pending, and it allowed the collective to resume cultivation.

Although it lasted for only a few months in 2003, this was a landmark victory for medical marijuana patients that few people are aware of, and WAMM became the only 100-percent federally legal medical marijuana garden to ever grow in America. During this period of jubilant celebration WAMM held a parade in downtown Santa Cruz, where members carried live cannabis plants fearlessly down the street.

I have seen firsthand how Valerie's leadership has transformed the lives of the seriously ill in truly extraordinary ways. WAMM's incredible strength lies in its community-based foundation, and together its members seem capable of miracles, but Valerie's leadership and vision made it all possible. Valerie has the gentleness of a kitten and the strength of a mountain lion. She's one of the most compassionate and heroic people I've ever met. Robert Anton Wilson, Ram Dass, and Nina Graboi have been members of WAMM, and they all praised Valerie's amazing work. Robert Anton Wilson said that "Valerie is simultaneously the most idealistic and the most practical person that I know."

On July 16 in Santa Cruz we celebrate WAMM/Medical Marijuana Day, which was officially declared a city holiday by Mayor Mike Rotkin in 2005. (Some of the other officially declared holidays in my beloved town of Santa Cruz include Ram Dass Day on November 7 and Robert Anton Wilson Day on July 23rd.) I'm convinced that one day there will be a statue of Valerie holding a raised cannabis flower toward the heavens in downtown Santa Cruz. To find out more about WAMM see www.wamm.org.

The cannabis plant has so many potential medicinal benefits that I'm sure entire research institutes of the future will be devoted to its study and that cannabis therapeutics will be a booming industry. Cannabis is so interesting and so controversial on a medical level because it really brings the mind/body connection mystery to the forefront. The active components in the cannabis plant, known as cannabinoids, which bind to receptors in the body and brain, do have measurable medical actions as anti-inflammatory, antinausea, antiseizure, antispasmodic, and antioxidant agents, but the benefits of some medically active cannabinoids blur curiously into the realm of mind.

Cannabis use moves the blood flow to different parts of the brain, for instance increasing blood flow into the right hemisphere, changing the way we think, shifting our perceptions, improving our sense of humor, and elevating our mood. These mental changes appear to be an inseparable component in why cannabis helps to make people feel better when they are faced with the end of their lives. When I interviewed Valerie she said:

> Many people have reported to me that marijuana has affected the way they look at their death. They tell me it has opened a door for them, or even a peephole, to allow them to accept death more willingly. There is nothing more important in this life than to be able to court death as a lover, to change our view and dance with her. This is our most profound opportunity.

I suspect that one additional reason why the more potent psychedelics can be so helpful in easing the dying process is because they give us a genuine glimpse of what really does happen to our consciousness after physical death. Nonetheless, what happens to consciousness after our material bodies decay and dissolve is a mystery—one of the biggest—and it's something that I've pondered for as long as I can remember. So I asked almost everyone I've interviewed what they thought about this timeless mystery.

WHAT HAPPENS TO US AFTER WE DIE?

What awaits us after the physical demise of our bodies? What will happen to you and me after we die? What happens to consciousness after the physical death of any living organism? From where does consciousness arise? Is consciousness an emergent property of complex information-processing systems, like brains, nervous systems, and possibly computers, or can it exist independent of a physical structure? Is everything conscious, as many mystics believe? This is one of the most ancient of all philosophical debates, and the question of what happens to consciousness after death is a recurring theme in my interviews.

To this day I'm continuously surprised by encounters with dogmatic scientists and religious believers who are convinced that they know for sure what happens. I don't think that anyone alive knows—not our smartest neuroscientists or our most highly achieved Buddhist lamas—although many of us certainly have our suspicions, some based on religious beliefs, and some on personal experiences with near-death states of consciousness, meditation, or psychedelics.

Death—what Terence McKenna called the black hole of biology—is, perhaps, the greatest mystery known to human beings. While there is compelling evidence that consciousness survives death and there is compelling evidence that it does not, the truth is no one knows for sure what happens when we die. I would be highly suspect of anyone who tells you otherwise.

Although the postbiological fate of human consciousness is a truly magnificent mystery, beliefs about what happens to consciousness after death generally fall into four traditional categories: reincarnation, eternal Heaven or Hell, union with God, or complete nonexistence. This limited range of possibilities is likely due to our strong fear of death, which creates a powerful emotional charge and makes playful speculation on this topic difficult for most people.

But if our fears can be suspended or transcended, and we can set our hopes and expectations aside, how might we explore this mystery and come up with alternative possibilities? Is it possible, as some people claim, that altered or mystical states of consciousness can give us insight into what happens after death? I think so.

Psychiatric researcher Stanislav Grof also thinks that his psychedelic experiences shed some light on what happens to consciousness after death. He said to me:

I have had experiences in my psychedelic sessions—quite a few of them—when I was sure I was in the same territory that we enter after death. In several of my sessions, I was absolutely certain that it had already happened and I was surprised when I came back.

However, when I asked neuroscientist John C. Lilly if his experiences with psychedelics influenced his perspective on what happens to human consciousness after biological death, he replied:

I refuse to equate my experiences with death. I think it's too easy to do that. When I was out for five days and nights on PCP, the guides took me to planets that were being destroyed and so on. I think ECCO [the Earth Coincidence Control Office] made me take that PCP so they could educate me. They kept hauling me around, and I tried to get back, but they said, "Nope, you haven't seen all the planets yet." One was being destroyed by atomic energy of war, one was being destroyed by a big asteroid that hit the planet, another one was being destroyed by biological warfare, and on and on and on. I realized that the universe is effectively benign; it may kill you but it will teach you something in the process.

A lot of the people I interviewed genuinely believe that some aspect of our consciousness survives death. Physician and spiritual teacher Deepak Chopra told me:

Nothing happens to consciousness after the death of the body. When two people are speaking on the phone and the lines are cut off, nothing happens to them. If the room I'm sitting in is destroyed, nothing happens to the space I'm in. Consciousness just loses a vehicle to express itself. If I destroy my radio set the broadcast is still happening, but it's not being actualized in the physical form, because the instrument is missing. So I think that when the instrument gets destroyed, consciousness ceases to express itself in the realm of space-time and causality, until it finds another vehicle to express itself. And, after a sufficient period of incubation, it does do that, by taking a quantum leap of creativity.

Spiritual teacher Ram Dass told me that he once asked Emmanuel, an entity that supposedly speaks through a woman named Pat Roderghas, what to tell people about dying, and he said, "Tell them it's absolutely safe. . . . Death is like taking off a tight shoe." So I asked Ram Dass what he thought happens to consciousness after death. He replied:

I think it jumps into a body of some kind, on some plane of existence, and it goes on doing that until it is with God. From a Hindu point of view, consciousness keeps going through reincarnations, which are learning experiences for the soul. I think what happens after you die is a function of the level of evolution of the individual. I think that if you have finished your work and you're just awareness that happens to be in a body, when the body ends it's like selling your Ford—it's no big deal. I suspect that some beings go unconscious. They go into what Christians call purgatory. They go to sleep during that process before they project into the next form. Others I think go through and are aware they are going through it, but are still caught. All the Bardos in the Tibetan Book of the Dead are about how to avoid getting caught. Those beings are awake enough for them to be collaborators in the appreciation of the gestalt in which their incarnations are flowing. They sort of see where they're coming from and where they're going. They are all part of the design of things. So, when you say, did you choose to incarnate? At the level at which you are free, you did choose. At the level at which you are not, you didn't. Then there are beings who are so free that when they go through death they may still have separateness. They may have taken the bodhisattva vow which says, "I agree to not give up separateness until everybody is free," and they're left with that thought. They don't have anything else. Then the next incarnation will be out of the intention to save all beings and not out of personal karma. That one bit of personal karma is what keeps it moving. To me, since nothing happened anyway, it's all an illusion—reincarnation and everything—but within the relative reality in which that's real, I think it's quite real.

Environmental activist John Robbins, author of *Diet for a New America,* answered my query about what happens after we die in two simple words:

It celebrates!

When I asked visionary artist Alex Grey what he thought happens to consciousness after death he replied:

I accept the near-death research and Tibetan Bardo explanations. Soon after physical death, when the senses shut down, you enter into the realms of light and archetypal beings. You have the potential to realize the clear light, our deepest and truest identity, if you recognize it as the true nature of your mind and are not freaked out. If you don't, you may contact other less appealing dimensions. No one can know, of course, until they get there. Some people have had experiences which give them certainty, but consciousness is the ultimate mystery. I'd like to surrender to the process on its deepest level when death occurs, but I will probably fail, and be back to interview you in the next lifetime.

Physicist Peter Russell, author of *The Global Brain,* answered my question "What do you think happens to consciousness after death?" by saying:

I have no idea. I've studied the near-death experience a bit, and it fascinates me. It would seem that one way of understanding it is that the individual consciousness is dissolving back into the infinite consciousness. The consciousness that I experience has this individual limitation because it is functioning in the world through my body, through my nervous system, through my eyes and ears. That's where our sense of being a unique individual comes from. When we begin to die and let go of our attachment to the body, consciousness lets go of that identity which it gained from its worldly functioning, and reconnects with a greater infinite identity. Those who've had near-death experiences often report there seems to be this dissolving of the senses, and a moving into light. Everything becomes light. There's this sense of deep peace and infinite love. Then they come to a threshold, beyond which there is no return. But we don't know what happens beyond there because the people who come back haven't gone beyond it. When I think of my consciousness, when I think of "me-ness," it seems to be something that is created during this life through this interaction with the world, but doesn't exist as an independent thing. I think that a lot of our concerns about death come from wanting to know what is going to happen to this "me" consciousness. Is "me" going to survive? I believe that this thing we call "me" is not going to survive. It's a temporary working model that consciousness uses, but in the end it's going to dissolve. A lot of our fear of death is that we fear this loss of "me-ness," this loss of a sense of a separate unique identity. It's interesting that people who've been through the near-death experiences and experienced this dissolving of the ego and realized that everything is okay when that happens, generally lose their fear of death. They feel incredible liberation in life.

I asked neuroscientist Candace Pert, who discovered the opiate receptor in the human brain, what she thinks happens to consciousness after death. She replied:

That's a great question. Years ago I had to answer that question to get a big honorarium, so I participated, and what I said then is still relevant. It's this idea that information is never destroyed. More and more information is constantly being created, and it's not lost, and energy and matter are interconvertible. So somehow there must be some survival, because one human being represents a huge amount of information. So I can imagine that there is survival, but I'm not sure exactly what form that it takes. I think Buddhist practice is interesting. There's this whole idea that you're actually preparing yourself for death, and if you do it just right you can make the transition better.

I asked celebrated stage magician Jeff McBride what he thought happens to consciousness after the death of the body. He replied:

I can't explain it, but I've seen it. It's a painting by Alex Grey in his first book, *Sacred Mirrors*. It's "Death," and the man laying there in bed, with his spirit ascending, twisting, and turning into the Net of Indra. It can't be put into language. But visionary artists like Alex Grey can paint it, and it is there for us to see. Consciousness in its unexplainable form survives, yes, but whether the ego remains, I would say no.

I asked physician Bernie Siegel, author of *Love, Medicine, and Miracles,* what he thought happens to consciousness after death. He said:

What I am sure happens to consciousness after death is that it continues on. I don't see it in a sense of saying, "Oh, I'm going to be reincarnated." No, your body is gone, but what you have experienced and are aware of will go on. So somebody will be born with your consciousness, and it will affect the life they live. I know people who see life's difficulties as a burden and say, "Why is God punishing me?" and "Why am I going through this?" Maybe these people ought to be asking "What am I here to learn, experience, and change?" Rather than sitting there whining and complaining. "What can I do?" and "What am I here to learn?" Now, I don't criticize these people because I remember Elisabeth Kübler-Ross saying that if you're in high school you don't get mad at somebody in first grade. So I think we're at different levels of consciousness based upon our experience and what we are born with. But I personally believe from my experience, for instance, that one of the reasons I'm a surgeon in this life is because I did a lot of destruction with a sword in a past life—killing people and animals. This is not conscious, like the answers I gave you earlier, but at a deeper level I chose to use a knife in this life to cure and heal with rather than kill with. I often say to people, "Think about things that affect you emotionally, that you have no explanation for. This may be due to some past-life experience, and that is why you're acting the way you're acting." Now, whether I'm right or wrong, I have to say that, as long as it's therapeutic that's what I'm interested in. But on a personal level, I believe that consciousness is nonlocal, and it can be carried on and picked up by people. I think this shows in animals too. There's a certain wisdom that they have.

When I asked physician Larry Dossey, author of *Healing Words: The Power of Prayer,* what he thought about this timeless mystery, he said:

If we acknowledge that consciousness is nonlocal—that it's infinite in space and time—then this really opens up all sorts of possibilities for the survival of consciousness following physical death. If you reason through this and follow the implications of these studies, you begin to realize that consciousness that's nonlocal and unrestricted in time is immortal. It's eternal. This is as hopeful as the current view of the fate of consciousness is dismal. This totally reverses things. So we are led to a position, I think, where we see that even though the body will certainly die, the most essential part of who we are can't die, even if it tried—because it's nonlocally distributed through time and space. Our grim vision of the finality of death is revised. Death is no longer viewed as a gruesome annihilation or the total destruction of all that we are. So there are tremendous spiritual implications that flow from these considerations, in addition to the implications for health. In fact, I believe that the implications for health are the least of it. A lot of people who encounter this area take a practical, bare-bones, utilitarian approach to it. They say, "Wow, now we've got a nifty new item in our black bag—a new trick to help people become healthier. Certainly these studies do suggest that this is a proper use of healing intentions and prayer, and I'm all for that, but the thing that really gets my juices flowing is the implication of this research for immortality. For me, that's the most exciting contribution of this entire field. The fear of death has caused more pain and suffering for human beings throughout history than all the physical diseases combined. The fear of death is the big unmentionable—and this view of consciousness is a cure for that disease, that fear of death.

Medical researcher Rick Strassman's book *DMT: The Spirit Molecule* makes a convincing case for the possibility that endogenous DMT in our brains helps to usher our souls in and out of our bodies. So I was especially interested in hearing what he thought happens to consciousness after death. He said:

I think it continues, but in some unknown form. I think a lot depends upon the nature of our consciousness during our lives—how attached to various levels of consensus reality it is. My late/former Zen teacher used to use the analogy of a lightbulb, with electric current passing through it. The lightbulb goes out, but the current continues, "changed" in a way, for its experience in the bulb. He also referred to like gravitating toward like in terms of the idea of the need for certain aspects of consciousness to develop further, before it can return to its source. That is, doglike aspects of our consciousness end up in a dog, humanlike aspects get worked through in another human, plantlike aspects into plants, and so on.

When I asked psychologist Dean Radin, who has done groundbreaking research into psychic phenomena, what he thought happens after we die, he said:

I expect that what we think of as ourselves—which is primarily personality, personal history, personality traits, and that sort of thing—goes away, because most of that information is probably contained in some way in the body itself. But as to some kind of a primal awareness, I think it probably continues, because it's not clear to me that that's produced by the body. In fact, I think that elementary awareness may be prior to matter. So when you go into a deep meditation and you lose your sense of personality, that may be similar to what it might be like to be dead. On the other hand, if you're not practiced at being in that deep state, or don't know how to pay attention to subtle variations in what might at first appear to be nothingness, it's not clear that your consciousness would stay around very long. In other words, you might have a momentary time when you have this sense of awareness, and then it just dissolves. It goes back and becomes part of the rest of everything. So it's like a drop that settles into the ocean and disappears into it. On the other hand, some people who either spend a lifetime preparing in meditation, or who are naturally adept, may be able to sustain being a drop. They may be able to settle into that ocean and still have a sense of their "dropness," even though they're also now part of the ocean. Then maybe one's sense of awareness would expand dramatically, and yet still have a sense of unity. I imagine that all this probably occurs in a state that is not bound by space and time as we normally think about it. So, presumably, you would have access to everything, everywhere. I imagine that something like that is the reason why ideas of reincarnation have come about, because people remember something about it. They may even remember something about the process of coming out of this ocean into a drop, into a particular incarnation, because a drop is embodied in a sense. . . . If there's anything that psychology teaches it's that people are different. So I imagine that there may be as many ways of experiencing after-death as there are people to experience it. And no one explanation is the "correct" one.

I asked quantum physicist Nick Herbert what he thought happens to consciousness after death. He replied:

I don't think it's possible for our type of consciousness to exist without matter around. But it needn't be this kind of matter in your brain. Different minds, different highs. The kind of practice we humans know about is taking possibilities and making them actual. You've got to have a universe to make them actual in. So we probably need matter then. It seems that our kind of consciousness and matter are inseparable. So that, when I die, probably most of my consciousness dies with me, because it's an interaction between the big mind, the big possibilities, and the small range of possibilities allotted to human bodies. But I may change my mind. I've been reading Ian Stevenson's book *Twenty Cases Suggestive of Reincarnation,* where little kids, when they begin to talk, say, "You're not my mother and dad. My parents live in this other town about four miles away." Then they begin giving

details about who their brothers and sisters are. It's very spooky stuff
. . . it certainly stretches your idea of what the mind is capable of, no
matter what explanation you have. So I may have to revise my ideas.
I would not believe in that ordinarily. I was perfectly willing to say
that my individuality dies with my body. There might be a large mind
that goes on, but this small mind probably dies with the body—the
memories and that sort of thing. That's what I would have said before
reading this book. I had always dismissed reincarnation as wrong. But
Stevenson's book is very persuasive. He describes just twenty cases, but
he has six hundred cases of more or less validity. And, of course, if
any one of those cases is true, it would invalidate the notion that consciousness dies with the body.

A few of the people didn't really have much to say on the matter
of what happens to consciousness after death. I asked anthropologist
Jeremy Narby, author of *The Cosmic Serpent,* what he thought happened to us after our bodies dissolve, and he enigmatically said to me:

In brief, I don't know, but I hope to see you at the bar.

When I asked biochemist and longevity researcher Aubrey de Grey,
author of *Ending Aging,* about the mystery of death, he said to me:

I have absolutely no opinion on that, and furthermore I don't intend
to do the experiment.

Some of the other people I interviewed had strong doubts that our
consciousness experiences any type of continued existence after we die.
When I asked linguist and political commentator Noam Chomsky
what he thought happened to consciousness after death he said:

I assume it's finished. That's the end. Death is the end of the organism, and the end of everything associated with it.

I asked comedian Paul Krassner what he thought happens to consciousness after death. He replied:

Oh, I think it dies with your physical body. That's my belief, and it's a pretty basic belief. It's like a Philip Wiley story, where an angel falls down from the sky, in front of this Air Force major, and he has to change his philosophy. So if I believed that, that my consciousness survived after my physical body died, I would have to change my philosophy.

When I asked Nobel Prize–winning chemist Kary Mullis, who helped to make genetic engineering possible, what he thought happens to consciousness after death, he said:

I think that consciousness decays to nothing after death. My approach is to ask myself, What do I have evidence for? It seems like every living process does end at some point. It's a fuzzy thing, but as your body dies, I think your consciousness probably dies with it. Now, that's what I think—but what I would like to believe might be different from that. I'm not absolutely certain that that's a question that I have enough evidence to answer. In science you're supposed to have evidence. It's all right to have a hypothesis, but you still have to have some evidence. You need to have something, like an indication, to make the hypothesis more than just a wish. Of course, being a scientist doesn't mean you don't have wishes. But, from a scientific point of view, I would say consciousness is definitely associated with the body as we know it. There's no reason to make up stories about things that we don't know anything about. However, when I'm thinking about what's possible, then anything is possible. I think it would be pretty neat if we didn't dissolve after our death. It's not a question that there is an answer for. There's no reason to think that consciousness continues after death, besides just the fact that we would like it, and that we don't want to dissolve—but that's not really a reasonable kind of a scientific premise. You couldn't get a National Science Foundation grant to study it properly, because we don't have any kind of indication that consciousness survives death. There are a lot of people who think that consciousness continues after we die, but I don't think that is reason for the scientist part of me to give it any truck at all. But there is a part of me, just like the rest of those people, that feels immortal and would like it to be that way. That question does not really have a rational answer. . . . If you were to take a vote around the planet, it would definitely come out that we are eternal and responsible somehow for ourselves and our actions forever. But that's not a rational point of view. There's nothing that we accept like that in science except for mathematical truths. The universe itself, we would say it changes, and it has a lifetime. And at some point, it will either return to a singularity, or it will just expand itself out of existence, or whatever. I mean, there's nothing around us that has that property of being immortal.

When I asked science-fiction author Bruce Sterling what he thought happens to consciousness after we die, he replied simply:

There isn't any. It's like going to sleep and not waking up.

A number of the people I interviewed answered my question about what happens to consciousness after death with skeptical but imaginative speculation. I asked science writer Clifford Pickover what he thought happens to human consciousness after our bodies perish. He replied:

If we believe that human consciousness is a product of the living brain, then consciousness evaporates when our brains die. When you fall asleep at night, consciousness seems to disappear, and then comes back upon awakening or when dreaming. If so, perhaps consciousness disappears when an individual dies as it does when a person enters nondreaming sleep. Someday, we may prevent this death by uploading our minds to machines, so in that sense our consciousness will survive brain death. I have nonreligious friends who speculate that consciousness exists as some kind of fundamental property of space-time, and I know of people who take DMT and who become certain that consciousness survives our bodily deaths, but of course all of this is speculation. If we believe that consciousness is the results of patterns of neurons in the brain, our thoughts, emotions, and memories could be replicated in moving assemblies of Tinkertoys. The Tinkertoy mind would have to be very big to represent the complexity of our minds, but still it could be done, in the same way people have made sophisticated computers out of Tinkertoys. In principle, our minds could be hypostatized in the patterns of twigs, in the movements of leaves, or in the flocking of birds. In any case, I believe that we all live happy lives, coded in the endless digits of π. Recall that the digits of π (in any base) not only go on forever but seem to behave statistically like a sequence of uniform random numbers. This means that somewhere inside the endless digits of π is a very close representation for all of us—the atomic coordinates of all our atoms, our genetic code, all our thoughts, all our memories. Given this fact, all of us are alive, and hopefully happy, in π. Pi makes us live forever. We all lead virtual lives in π. We are immortal.

Surprisingly, the late guitarist for the Grateful Dead, Jerry Garcia, initially told me that he didn't think that consciousness continues after death. He told me:

It probably dies with the body. Why would it exist apart from the body?

I said to Jerry that many people have had convincing near-death experiences, where they felt like they were able to exist independently their body. He said:

> That's true. But unfortunately the only ones who have gone past that are still dead. I don't know what consciousness is apart from a physical being. I once slipped out of my body accidentally. I was at home watching television and I slid out through the soles of my feet. All of a sudden I was hovering up by the ceiling, looking down at myself. So I know that I can disembody myself somehow from my physical self, but more than that I have no way of knowing. . . . [Reincarnation] may happen in a very large way. It may be that part of all the DNA coding, the specific memory, returns. There's definitely information in my mind that did not come from this lifetime. Not only is there some, but there's tons of it! Enormous, vast reservoirs. Dreams are kind of a clue. What are these organizing principles that make it so you experience these realities that are emotionally as real as this life is? You can feel grief or be frightened in a dream just as badly as you can in this life. And the psychedelic experience is similar in that it has the power to convince you of its authenticity. It's hard to ignore that once you have experienced it.

Jerry Garcia had a very strange and utterly fascinating near-death experience that he shared with me. It reminded me of a DMT trip. Jerry said:

> My main experience was one of furious activity and tremendous struggle in a sort of futuristic spaceship vehicle with insectoid presences. After I came out of my coma, I had this image of myself as these little hunks of protoplasm that were stuck together kind of like stamps with perforations between them that you could snap off. They were run through with neoprene tubing, and there were these

insects that looked like cockroaches, which were like message units that were kind of like my bloodstream. That was my image of my physical self, and this particular feeling lasted a long time. It was really strange . . . it lasted a couple of days! It . . . gave me a greater admiration for the incredible baroque possibilities of mentation. The mind is so incredibly weird. The whole process of going into coma was very interesting too. It was a slow onset—it took about a week—and during this time I started feeling like the vegetable kingdom was speaking to me. It was communicating in comic dialect in iambic pentameter. So there were these Italian accents and German accents, and it got to be this vast gabbling. Potatoes and radishes and trees were all speaking to me. It was really strange. It finally just reached hysteria, and that's when I passed out and woke up in the hospital.

One of my very favorite responses to the question of what might happen to consciousness after death came from Terence McKenna, who said:

I've thought about it. When I think about it I feel like I'm on my own. The Logos doesn't want to help here, has nothing to say to me on the subject of biological death. What I imagine happens is that for the self time begins to flow backward; even before death, the act of dying is the act of reliving an entire life, and at the end of the dying process, consciousness divides into the consciousness of one's parents and one's children, and then it moves through these modalities, and then divides again. It's moving forward into the future through the people who come after you, and backward into the past through your ancestors. The further away from the moment of death it is, the faster it moves, so that after a period of time, the Tibetans say forty-nine days, one is reconnected to everything that ever lived, and the previous ego-pointed existence is defocused, and one is, you know, returned to the ocean, the morphogenetic field, or the One of Plotinus—you choose your term. A person is a focused illusion of being, and death occurs when the illusion of being can be sustained no longer. Then everything flows out and away from this disequilibrium state that life is. It is a state of disequilibrium, and it is maintained for decades, but finally, like all disequilibrium states, it must yield to the second law of thermodynamics, and at that point it runs down, its specific character disappears into the general character of the world around it. It has returned then to the void/plenum.

Terence McKenna was the first person I interviewed, and he was the first person I formally asked the question of what happens to consciousness after death. That was in 1988. Twenty years later, in 2008, I asked his brother, pharmacologist Dennis McKenna, the same question. He replied:

Oh, boy. I don't know, and I don't think that anybody does. I think that's the only honest answer anybody can give—no matter what they may claim. Whether people claim to know or not, the bottom line is nobody really knows. Now, I can speculate a lot. I think that the basis for speculation revolves around the question of whether consciousness is something that resides in the brain. The question is whether consciousness is something that is generated mainly by the brain and the neural activity of the brain, or whether consciousness is something more like the ether and something that permeates the space-time continuum. In other words, is the brain more like a generator or a detector? The brain could be like a radio antennae, essentially, and you change the channel. You change the frequency of the radio antennae and you pick up different stations. It could be that the brain is more like a radio tuner for something that's everywhere in the continuum. I think if that's what consciousness is, then the idea that it persists after death is certainly much more plausible. If that's true, then that's not even the correct way to interpret the question. Maybe asking if consciousness persists after death is like asking, Does the electromagnetic spectrum persist after you break the radio and send it to the trash heap? Of course it does, because it has nothing to do with the individual radio receiver. It's still out there. So if you choose to believe that—and I don't think we really know yet what it is—then I think there's every possibility that in some sense consciousness does persist after death, or some nucleus, or a kernel of individual consciousness reemerges into the universal mind or whatever you want to call it. Certainly this is many people's experiences on psychedelics, that they have this type of experience, and that convinces them that that's what happens after death. I think that if there's a pharmacological analog for the death experience, I think psychedelics are it, especially DMT. Rick Strassman's work very strongly suggests that DMT may play this role. We know that DMT exists in the human brain, and that it may have important functions at certain stages of development—one of them being at the moment of death. The stressers that are expressed on the organism and on the brain at the moment of death may cause a massive release of DMT and other neural chemicals in the brain that, in some sense, simulates the near-death experience, or actually is the near-death experience. Do you pass through the doorway and get beyond that, to some sort of Pleroma, where all minds are merged together? I mean, hell, I don't know. It's not an implausible idea.

Being the philosopher that Timothy Leary was, I had imagined that he spent a good deal of his time when he was dying pondering what his afterlife might be like. When I interviewed Timothy for my first interview book *Mavericks of the Mind* in 1989, one of the questions that I asked him was what he thought happened to consciousness after the death of the body. He never really answered the question and went off on this whole rap about cryonic suspension. In 1996 when Timothy was actually dying, I thought he would be more apt to speak about his views on the post-death experience.

However, when I interviewed Timothy again he continued to evade the question, saying that he always tried to be "scientific," and that people can have done to their bodies whatever they like after they die. "It can be cremation, it can be worms," he said. Nonetheless, this time I was much more persistent with my questioning, and I did finally manage to get something out of him. Because Timothy mentioned only what would happen to his body, I asked him if he thought that his consciousness could exist independently of his body. He replied:

Sure. Oh, absolutely. Of course . . . Well, I've taken a lot of LSD. . . . Many times I'd feel my leather hands, and there's no warm blood inside them. Flesh has become simulated skin. Yeah, I've been there.

Two of my favorite answers to the question of what happens to consciousness after death came from Robert Anton Wilson, who answered the question for me twice. The first was in 1989, when he said:

Somebody asked a Zen master, "What happens after death?" He replied, "I don't know." And the querent said, "But you're a Zen master!" He said, "Yes, but I'm not a dead Zen master." Somebody asked Meister Eckart, the great German mystic, "Where do you think you'll go after death?" He said, "I don't plan to go anywhere." Those are the best answers I've heard so far. My hunch is that consciousness is a nonlocal function of the universe as a whole, and our brains are only local transceivers. As a matter of fact, it's a very strong hunch, but I'm not going to dogmatize about it.

The second time was in 2005, when Wilson said:

I haven't died yet, so I can't speak with any assurance about that. My guesses remain guesses. I grant equal respect to the opinions of all men, women, and ostriches, but no matter how sure any of them sound, I still suspect them of guessing, just like me. I wish they would use that liberating word "maybe" more often in their speculations. If I must flounder around in metaphysics, "the great Serbonian bog where armies whole have sunk," I know of only five possibilities: (1) Heaven, (2) Hell, (3) reincarnation, (4) union with God or some other entity a lot like God, and (5) oblivion. Only Heaven seems frightening to me; an eternity of "bliss" with nobody around but Christians—such messmates as Pat Robertson, Jerry Falwell, and others of that ilk— really sounds awful. There's even a sinister rumor that the streets are guarded (brrrrrr!) by the United States Marines. Fortunately, according to the leading proponents of this model, I can't get sent there because I don't believe in Christ. Oh, goody. Of course, Hell sounds almost as bad, but it has its good points. Everybody I admire from all history will get sent there, so the conversation should prove lively and stimulating. Besides, I find it impossible to believe that "God" (i.e., the assumed "Mind" behind the universe) suffers from the kind of sadistic psychosis necessary to delight in eternal torture, and if He (or She or It) does have that kind of nasty streak, well, as a part-time Buddhist, I'll just have to forgive Him (or Her or It). I've started practicing for this eventuality by forgiving all the people who've made this planet a good simulation of Hell.

The reincarnation model seems cheerier and somewhat less goofy than these morbid notions, so it doesn't bother me. I even wish I could believe in it. Union with God seems a great idea to me, if I understand it, like an acid trip that never ends. Now that's what I'd prefer, if I have any choice in the matter. Finally, there's the oblivion model. I've never understood why so many people, like Woody Allen, find oblivion totally dreadful. If you're oblivious, that implies no experience and, of course, no experiencer either. How can you fear or even resent what you will never experience? It seems to me that only an advanced case of narcissism, or a mangled confusion of the map with the territory, can explain the bum rap that oblivion gets from most people. We all go there every night, between dreams, and it doesn't hurt at all.

Robotic expert Hans Moravec, author of *Mind Children,* proposed a multiple universe theory to explain what he thought happens to consciousness after death. When I interviewed him, he said:

> In the space of all possible worlds, there are certainly going to be continuations of consciousness in some of them, no matter what happens to us. . . . No matter how we die, in some possible world there's a way in which we, through some mechanism or other, continue on.

I asked inventor Ray Kurzweil what he thinks happens to human consciousness after biological death. He replied:

> That's a question that really is beyond our current understanding. I do talk about some dilemmas in our understanding of consciousness. For example, is there a continuity of consciousness even in biological human life that continues? Am I the same consciousness that Ray Kurzweil was a year ago? And you say, "Well, Ray, you're the same stuff. It's the same arm and the same face." But, actually, no, I'm completely different particles than I was a year ago. Virtually all of my cells have been replaced. Now you say, "Well, okay. But, Ray, most of your neurons haven't been replaced. Some of them have, but neurons tend to last longer than most of the other cells, which get turned over. But even those neurons that existed a year ago actually were made of different particles. The actual physical atoms and molecules making them up have been replaced, so nothing is the same as it was a year ago. Actually the only thing that's the same is the pattern. There's a certain continuity of pattern, of how all these atoms and molecules are put together, that does have a continuity between myself today and myself a year ago. So that means what we are is a pattern, and the pattern persists. I draw an analogy to the pattern that water makes in a stream, as it, say, darts around some rocks.

If you look at a stream going around some rocks, you see a certain pattern, and that pattern can look very stable. It can stay the same for hours or even years. But the actual water molecules making up the pattern change in a fraction of a second, because water's flowing by. So it's completely different stuff every fraction of a second. But the pattern stays the same.

And we're really pretty much like that pattern of water, because this stuff is flowing through us, and we're not the same particles at all. So if you hold your arm and say, "Well this is me," it's not. We're just a pattern. And what is a pattern? A pattern is information. It's knowledge. I think that there's a great loss of pattern in death, a great loss of knowledge and information. I think death is a tragedy. And I think that, because we've had no alternative up until now, people have gone to great lengths to rationalize death, saying, "Oh, well. Death really isn't such a bad thing, and death's really a wonderful thing. It's really elevating and we transcend." We've gone to tremendous efforts to rationalize what's obviously a terrible thing and a profound loss, so that we think it's really a good thing. Well, I don't think it's a good thing. I think death is a tragedy. I think it's a tragedy at the age of ninety just as much as if it's at the age of ten or twenty. And I think we're now reaching a point where we can do something about it. We don't have the technologies in hand at this moment, to, say, just do X, Y, and Z, and you can live indefinitely, but we do have technologies in health understanding that can keep us healthy until we get the next bridge, which is the full flowering of the biotechnology revolution. This will not allow us to live forever, but will be a bridge to the next revolution, which is the full flowering of the nanotechnology revolution, and that will allow us to live indefinitely by being able to really rebuild our bodies and brains using much more durable technologies. So we actually do have a path, which I call a bridge to a bridge to a bridge, that can give us virtual immortality.

My children's generation actually doesn't have to do a lot to take advantage of that, barring an unusual premature death. But by the time kids today who are twenty become forty these technologies will be at a fairly mature level. This is a message, though, for the baby boomer generation. I'm fifty-five, and my contemporaries, if they really go to the edge of what's known today in terms of health and medical knowledge, can stay alive and healthy until the full flowering of the biotechnology revolution, which will then keep them going longer till the flowering of the nanotechnology revolution. But I would say that 99.99 percent of my contemporaries are completely oblivious to this fact and are planning to just live and die the old-fashioned way. And they will be essentially the last generation to die in the normal course. Radical life extension is another one of the profound transformations that lies ahead.

Medical marijuana activist and WAMM cofounder Valerie Corral spends a lot of time with people who are dying. Valerie was with the late author Laura Huxley (Aldous Huxley's widow) on the night that she left this world, when she said to her, "Tell Ram Dass it's all brand new!" When I asked Valerie what she thought happens to consciousness after death, she first asked me to define the word *consciousness*. I said that I simply meant one's basic sense of self or awareness, one's sense of "I." After giving her this definition she replied:

Certainly not one thing. I don't think that one thing happens. I really feel like my experience of dissolving . . . [during a mystical experience at the age of fourteen] felt like the most natural thing. I would say that my observations lead me to think that it's kind of a dissolution, but I don't think there's a distinction between who I am and what I dissolve into. Will I still know that I'm dissolved after it happens? Will I know that I'm part of something greater? Will I feel that? I have. So that's what I think.

I asked the late physician Jack Kevorkian, who was imprisoned for years due to his practice of euthanasia, what he thought happens to consciousness after death. He replied:

> No living being in this world knows exactly and certainly—indeed even faintly—what absolute physical death is. One can only know that it occurred. Despite impressive philosophical and religious mythologizing, as well as the anecdotal bunkum called near-death experiences, nobody has ever survived absolute death. At present that survival would offer the only (but now inaccessible) means of gaining reliable and certain knowledge about it.

When I asked biologist Rupert Sheldrake, author of *A New Science of Life,* what he thought about this timeless mystery, he said:

> For me the best starting point for this question is experience. We all have the experience of a kind of alternative body when we dream. Everyone in their dreams has the experience of doing things that their physical body is not doing. When I dream I might be walking around, talking to people, even flying, yet these activities in my dreams, which happen in a body, are happening in my dream body. They're not happening in my physical body, because my physical body's lying down asleep in bed. So we all have a kind of parallel body in our dreams. Now, where exactly that's happening, what kind of space our dreams are happening in, is another question. It's obviously a space to do with the mind or consciousness, but we can't take for granted that that space is confined to the inside of the head. Normally people assume it must be, but they assume that all our consciousness is in our heads, and I don't agree with that assumption. I think our minds extend beyond our brains in every act of vision, something I discuss in my book *The Sense of Being Stared At, and Other Aspects of the Extended Mind.* So I think this, then, relates to out-of-the-body experiences, where

people feel themselves floating out of their body and see themselves from outside, or lucid dreams, where people in their dreams become aware they're dreaming and can will themselves to go to particular places by gaining control of their dream. These are, as it were, extensions of the dream body.

Now, when we die, it's possible, to my way of thinking, that it may be rather like being in a dream from which we can't wake up. This realm of consciousness that we experience in our dreams may exist independent of the brain, because it's not really a physical realm. It's a realm of possibility or imagination. It's a realm of the mind. It's possible that we could go on living in a kind of dream world, changing and developing in that world, in a way that's not confined to the physical body. Now, whether that happens or not is another question, but it seems to me possible. The out-of-body experiences and the near-death experiences may suggest that's indeed what's going to happen to us when we die. But the fact is that we're not really going to find out until we do die, and what happens then may indeed depend on our expectations. It may be that materialists and atheists who think death will just be a blank would actually experience a blank. It may be that their expectations will affect what actually happens. It may be that people who think they'll go to a heavenly realm of palm oases and almond-eyed dancing girls really will. It may be that the afterlife is heavily conditioned by our expectations and beliefs, just as our dreams are.

Sheldrake's response rings true for me, because it seems like so much of what we experience in life is deeply influenced by our beliefs. Why would death be any different?

I asked media theorist Douglas Rushkoff, author of *Media Virus!*, what he thought happens to consciousness after death. He replied:

I really have no idea. I would guess it goes on for a few minutes. You get to Heaven, and you have those great life-after-life experiences, and then . . . [Laughs] nothing! [Laughs] I would think the only way for a person to have anything approaching consciousness after death—real death, when the body actually stops metabolizing, or there's just no metabolic processes and the brain is really dead dead—would be, while that person is alive, to learn to identify so profoundly with something other than his or her own ego, so that when the self dies, the identification goes on. But most of us really believe in the illusion of individuality. We believe who we are is us. So, in a sense, it blows the question out of the water, finally, because you say, "Well, what happens to consciousness after death?" Well, what happens to your consciousness after someone else's death? Not a hell of a lot. I mean, you might feel bad that they died, but their consciousness is gone, except for the part of it that's now in everybody else. It certainly shouldn't be anybody's goal to extend consciousness after death, because that's still just a person trying to project their ego. But I would think a fringe benefit of developing true compassion for other people is that if you do identify with other people, other things, and other systems—things that are beyond the four walls of your own limited personal consciousness—then the death of you or me is inconsequential. But I think that for 99.9999 percent of people the chances are that they just die. . . . I would think that the only way out would be to get out while you're here. I don't think you can get out after you're dead.

When I asked lucid dream researcher Stephen LaBerge what he thought about the survival of consciousness after death, he said:

Let's suppose I'm having a lucid dream. The first thing I think is, "Oh, this is a dream. Here I am." Now, the "I" here is who I think Stephen is. Now, what's happening, in fact, is that Stephen is asleep in bed somewhere, not in this world at all, and he's having a dream that he's in this room talking to you. With a little bit of lucidity I'd say, "This is a dream, and you're all in my dream." A little more lucidity and I'd know you're a dream figure and this is a dream-table, and this must be a dream-shirt and a dream-watch. And what's this? It's got to be a dream-hand. And, well, so what's this? It's a dream-Stephen! So a moment ago I thought this is who I am, and now I know that it's just a mental model of who I am. So reasoning along those lines, I thought, *I'd like to have a sense of what my deepest identity is, what's my highest potential, which level is the realest in a sense?*

With that in mind at the beginning of a lucid dream, I was driving in my sports car down through the green spring countryside. I see an attractive hitchhiker at the side of the road, thought of picking her up, but said, "No, I've already had that dream. I want this to be a representation of my highest potential." So the moment I had that thought and decided to forgo the immediate pleasure, the car started to fly into the air and the car disappeared and my body, also. There were symbols of traditional religions in the clouds, the Star of David and the cross and the steeple and Near Eastern symbols. As I passed through that realm, higher beyond the clouds, I entered into a vast emptiness of space that was infinite and it was filled with potential and love. And the feeling I had was, *This is home! This is where I'm from and I'd forgotten that it was here.* I was overwhelmed with joy about the fact that this source of being was immediately present, that it was always here, and I had not been seeing it because of what was in my way. So I started singing for joy with a voice that spanned three or four octaves and resonated with the cosmos with words like, "I praise thee, O Lord!" There wasn't any I, there was no thee, no Lord, no duality somehow, but sort of. *Praise be* was the feeling of it. My belief is that the experience I had of this void, that's what you get if you take away the brain. When I thought about the meaning of that, I recognized that the deepest identity I had there was the source of being, the all and nothing that was here right now, that was what I was too, in addition to being Stephen.

So the analogy that I use for understanding this is that we have these separate snowflake identities. Every snowflake is different in the same sense that each one of us is, in fact, distinct. So here is death, and here's the snowflake, and we're falling into the infinite ocean. So what do we fear? We fear that we're going to lose our identity, we'll be melted, dissolved in that ocean and we'll be gone. But what may happen is that the snowflake hits the ocean and feels an infinite expansion of identity and realizes, *What I was, in essence, was water!* So we're each one of these little frozen droplets and we feel only our individuality but not our substance, but our essential substance is common to everything in that sense, so now God is the ocean. So we're each a little droplet of that ocean, identifying only with the form of the droplet and not with the majesty and the unity. There may be intermediate states where, to press the metaphor, the seed crystal is recycled and makes another snowflake in a similar form or something like that, but that's not my concern. My concern is with the ocean—that's what I care about. So whether or not Stephen, or some deeper identity of Stephen, survives, well, that'd be nice if that were so. But how can one not be satisfied with being the ocean?

When I asked the late comedian George Carlin, whom I thought was one of the funniest human beings to ever exist, what he thought happens to consciousness after death, he said:

I don't know. It's obviously one of the most fascinating things that we don't know. I profess no belief in God, which, by definition, is true, especially if we take the accepted definition of God. But to be an atheist is to also have a belief and have a system, and I don't know that I like that either. And yet I shrink from the word *agnostic,* because it seems like a handy weigh station to park at. I don't know. And I'm satisfied not knowing, because it allows me to be filled with speculation and imagination about all the possibilities. I find it interesting to read about or listen to people who have highly developed beliefs in an afterlife—forgetting now Christians, God, and religion—and second chances, reincarnation, other planes of existence, other dimensions. Now we get into the physical realm of the universes, which is interesting because *universe* means "one," and here we are talking about multiuniverses. . . . I don't care what happens to me after I die, but I know this. I know that if there's some sort of moral reckoning, I know I'll come out clean. I know I've never done a mean thing intentionally to anyone. I know I've only tried to make people feel better and be more at ease. I don't mean professionally. I mean in personal relationships. I try to put people at ease, make them feel good. And I know that if there's some sort of reckoning by something that says, "Well, let's look at your record here," I'm clean. So I'm happy with that.

I once asked physicist Stephen Hawking about multiple universes. He often writes and lectures about multiple universes and baby universes. I asked him how there could be more than one universe, when, by definition, the word *universe* means "everything that exists." Hawking told me that a universe "is a set of related events." Apparently, you can have many self-contained sets of related events that have no influence on one another, and each one is considered its own universe. I told Carlin about this dialogue that I had with Hawking. Carlin said:

It's just fascinating, and you get lost in the possibilities. There's no way to hang your hat on any of these things. There's just no way to say, "Ah, this a good one. I'll go with this." Because they're all titillating, and they're tempting. And they're all entertaining to the way I've developed my mind. I find it highly entertaining to consider wormholes and alternate parallel universes and all the things that Robert Anton Wilson sometimes writes about. It's just endlessly entertaining and fascinating. So I'm quite content in being in this position. I think there's a certain arrogance of spirit that says, "Here's the way it goes. Here's what happens." Or to narrow it down to two things or so, maybe it's okay. I don't know. But for me, I can't live that way. I have to keep all the doors open, just for the fun of it.

I asked the late beat poet Allen Ginsberg, composer of the legendary poem "Howl," what he thought happens to human consciousness after biological death. He said:

I don't know. The Tibetans say that some kind of etheric electricity or some kind of impulse moves on. I think it's a good idea to cultivate an openness to the possibilities that might occur. When you're drowning, once you've stopped breathing, there's still about eight minutes of consciousness before brain death, and there have been people who have been resuscitated, so something is there. In that eight minutes, what should you prepare for? My meditation practices are on the breath, so then what happens after I stop breathing? I asked my guru this question and he started laughing. He said that was the purpose of the advanced meditation practices, the visualization, the mantra, the mandala, all that stuff. He said, "If I were you, I wouldn't pretend this or that, openness or emptiness. I would go along with whatever made the process more comfortable." As for what happens after death, I've always been a little skeptical about anything persevering. I think the process of dying takes over, whatever you think, and goes on automatic. What you think may be harmonious with what happens, but what happens is going to happen in any case. Sometimes I think that you enter open space and become open space. In the last moment you don't want to be pissed off, even if there's no rebirth. So it's a good idea to get into the frequency of some kind of meditative practice, in case there's no afterlife. In case there is, it's also a good idea. It prepares you for whatever situation. "Do not go gently into that good night. / Rage, rage against the dying of the light." You know that poem? It seems the worst advice possible. . . . I'm a little scared, yeah, but I'm not afraid to admit it.

I asked Allen what it was about death that frightened him. He said:

How about entering a realm where there's twenty-nine devils sticking red-hot pokers up my behind and into my feet? Maybe I'll turn into a big prick with this little tiny asshole. . . . [Nonexistence] wouldn't be so bad. It would be the fear of existing again in another life. Popping up again, like "Pop Goes the Weasel," and being stuck with whatever hard-on you started out with. You could have an obsession and think, *Oh, I should have cut that out long ago! I should have stopped lusting after pretty boys long ago!* You're born into a universe with nothing but pretty boys and you get stuck there for another hundred years until you realize, uh oh, you're going to die. Something like that. I'm not quite up to the adventure yet, but on the other hand . . .

I asked theologian Matthew Fox, author of *Original Blessing,* what he thought happens to human consciousness after biological death. He replied:

I don't think that any beauty is lost in the universe. Hildegard of Bingen says, "No warmth is lost in the universe." Einstein said, "No energy's lost." I think that the beauty hangs around. Rupert Sheldrake would call this the morphic resonance, and the Christian tradition would call it the Communion of Saints. The East might call it the incarnation. . . . Eckhart says, "When I return to the source, the core, the fountain of the Godhead, no one will ask what I've been doing. No one will have missed me." What he's really saying is that there's no judgment.

I asked the late psychedelic spokeswoman Nina Graboi, author of *One Foot in the Future,* what she thought happens to human consciousness after death. Her answer took on a much greater significance for me after she died, which I'll explain later in this chapter. Graboi responded to my inquiry by saying:

I know nothing about that except that my consciousness, when it is liberated from the body, goes into strange and unfathomable yet somehow familiar dimensions. The only certainty I came away with from my LSD studies is that I am not my body. Strangely enough, today many New Agers see this as heresy. They call it dualism. "I am what I eat. I and my body are one," they say. True, I'm no more separate from my body than from the air I breathe, or from a rock, or from a worm, or from anything at all. So I wind up in a cosmic goo. But we have learned to name things so we can distinguish between what's me and what's not me. I am not my body any more than I am the air, the rock, or the worm. I think of my body as my spacesuit, which I will discard once it has grown threadbare—but I will go on. People in our culture think of death as the enemy, yet death is as natural as eating. There are two possibilities: either we die and everything is over, we're just simply gone—so what's there to be afraid of? Or else life is a spiral that is eternally ascending. We may or may not come back to this planet in physical form, but I think that we are travelers, and that our journey is endless. I don't like the idea of being in pain and all that stuff that leads up to the actual death, but death itself doesn't frighten me.

I probed Reverend Ivan Stang, one of the principal founders of the Church of the SubGenius, for his thoughts about what happens to consciousness after death. He said:

I'll give you the most concrete answer you've perhaps ever gotten to that one: I don't have the slightest idea. And if I said that I did, I'd be one lying motherfucker. I saw your talk at the Starwood Festival, David, and you discussed some of the responses that you've gotten to that question from the people you've interviewed. You mentioned Jerry Garcia's believing that when you're dead, you're dead, which actually is what the scientific literature would definitely lead one to believe, for the most part.

On the other hand, I noticed that Dr. Timothy Leary never would give you a straight answer to that one. I would have to throw my vote in with Dr. Tim. That is a very interesting question. If we had a happy answer to it, about half of the world would probably commit suicide as soon as the bills came in. Except for there's that one catch: if you kill yourself, then you don't go to Heaven. But think about it evolutionarily. If we knew there was a life after death that would not be a very handy thing. I would imagine that the spirits, the angels, and the Gods would just as soon keep us guessing and paying lip service—which, obviously, most of them are. I've noticed that a lot of the people who talk the most about Heaven seem to me, behind it all, to be not at all that sure that that's the way things are going to happen. They're a lot more scared of death than I seem to be. I hate to see things wasted, but the last thing I'm scared of is death. In fact, I've already got my tombstone statement worked out. I've been telling this to people for years now. It should say, *Reverend Ivan Stang, born 1953, died, blah blah. Quote: "I'll get them for this."* That's about as wonderful a statement of futility as our war on God, which I now declare every time I do a sermon. I declare war on God—on the God that has to be defended from jerks like me by little illiterate old ladies, the God you have to clap your hands to believe in, or he'll dry up and blow away like Tinkerbell.

Although some of the people I interviewed responded to my query about the possibility of an afterlife in accordance with the four traditional views, and a few said that they just accepted the mystery, others entertained far-less-conventional notions. Exploring ideas about what happens after we die with these remarkable individuals only deepens the mystery of death, because it expands the range of possibilities. Although no one can be certain about evidence of an afterlife from near-death experiences, supposed spirit communications, psychedelic experiences, or spiritual revelations, contemplating the possibilities of a postdeath existence can not only be psychologically liberating and thought-provoking, it can deeply inspire the imagination.

There's lots of interesting and often compelling evidence that consciousness can exist independently of the brain and that it may survive death. Out-of-body experiences, near-death experiences, psychedelic experiences, reincarnation studies, and numerously documented spirit-contact experiences support this notion, as does a basis for their existence in quantum physics. If you're interested in these possibilities take a look at the brilliant work of Charles Tart, Sam Parnia, Ian Stevenson, and Stanislav Grof.

There's probably at least as much evidence to support the claim that consciousness can exist independently of the brain as there is evidence that consciousness is dependent on the brain. On the flip side, we can take a powerful sedative like a barbiturate that will completely obliterate our consciousness, and we seem to lose consciousness for a large portion of the time that we're asleep. So who really knows what happens? It's a serious mystery, and quantum field theory leaves open plenty of latitude for possible mechanisms that consciousness may survive bodily death.

When I asked psychologist Charles Tart, who has studied near-death experiences, what he thought happens after death, he replied:

After doing more than fifty years of professional work with consciousness now, one of the things that's really been interesting to me is that it's become more and more clear that there's an aspect of consciousness that appears to transcend physical or material reality. At the same time, it's also clear to me that a lot of our ordinary consciousness is very dependent on being shaped by the nature of our bodies, or at least by our brains. Clearly, that shaping is completely gone from one's reality after death. I was once asked what I thought about the evidence for survival after death, and I summed it up by saying this: when I die, I expect that I'll probably be unconsciousness for a bit—but I expect to recover from it. On the other hand, I'm not quite sure that the "I" that will recover from death will be the same "I" who dies. I think that there's going to be some major changes in whatever survives, and this is a gross generalization. There is a very large body of literature about the possibility that consciousness survives death, and I've been running a discussion group with many of the world's experts about this for years. The commonality of the NDE helped to decrease my bias against what I thought was an impossibility. However, I think that although consciousness probably survives death, it probably doesn't survive in quite the same form as we're used to. However, if people merely believe in an afterlife it may influence their interpretation of the evidence.

I asked Edgar Dean Mitchell, the lunar module pilot for NASA's *Apollo 14* space mission in 1971 and the sixth man to walk on the moon, what he thinks happens to consciousness after death. Mitchell reported a mystical experience in space, which I described in the introduction, and afterward founded the Institute of Noetic Sciences to study psychic and other unexplained phenomena. Mitchell said:

All I can do is state the evidence. Let me give you my position and my approach to this, because it's very important and germane. My take is that the universe is natural. It's a natural universe and therefore knowable. If Descartes was right, then the supernatural aspect of the universe is not knowable by humans; it's only knowable by God, if you will. Well, I reject that postulate. I'm a positivist in the sense of Karl Popper's investigation. We may not be able to prove things, but we have to advance by creating hypotheses and then try to falsify them. So I have made the single assumption in my work that the universe is natural and proceed, therefore, to try to understand consciousness in terms of that. That means it's knowable, and if we push on it we can gain understanding and data. Now, essentially, we have two major philosophies: science and theology. There's the materialist philosophy, which is science. Classic Newtonian physics believes that everything is based upon matter, and the interaction of molecules is deterministic. The other philosophy is the idealist, which is the basis of theology, and that believes that everything is consciousness, and that consciousness is independent of matter. If that is so, then it's assumed that the universe is unknowable. So I simply make the unitary assumption that the universe is knowable and natural, and to pursue and extend our science, of course we have to look at subjective phenomena. Then we will eventually get to the answer. And so far I haven't been wrong. Everything we approach seems to be right.

Now, to answer your question, does consciousness survive death? The modeling we can do so far does not accommodate that idea. It doesn't point in that direction. The most advanced modeling we can do at the moment, I believe, is called quantum holography, which I've been very forward in working with and pushing. Essentially it says that the historical events of all matter are preserved in its quantum holographic record, and it's preserved nonlocally, which means it is useful or usable by future generations. Now, there's a lot of *ifs*, *and*s, and *but*s that go with this, but this is the sound-bite version. So this supports the idea that information is there available to us at the psychic or subjective level, and it's rooted in this quantum holographic phenomena. But this does not suggest that consciousness can exist independently of the living system. It merely says the information is available to the living system. So there's a whole host of ramifications to this. It seems that this quantum holographic phenomenon is a mechanism for nonlocal information in nature. I've written a paper on this subject called "Nature's Mind: The Quantum Holograph." Others have picked up on it, and we're pushing it very hard. It seems to be responsible not only for psychic abilities, as we understand them, but also the basis of why we have perception at all. So the modeling, so far, suggests that information about existence is preserved following life. We haven't yet been able to account for discarnate consciousness. I don't know how to account for that or how to model that. That is an article of faith among a lot of religious people, but as a scientist I can't model that yet. Although I think we've made enormous progress in modeling much of psychic stuff, we haven't been able to model life after death.

I spoke with late psychiatric researcher John Mack, who was familiar with research that suggested the possibility of an afterlife, about what he thought happens to consciousness after death. He said:

The honest answer is, of course, I don't know. There are various reasons to believe that there is some continuation of consciousness after death from research that's been done on near-death experiences, and from certain people who, seemingly, have the capacity to enter into that realm and return—to live in both the realm where spirits reside and this realm and report upon it. I myself am involved in research that has to do with a colleague and friend who died a year and a half ago. She has been communicating with her husband, friends, and patients, in ways that leave, in my mind, little doubt it is she. In other words, there's information being communicated that only she had. Then there's a whole body of research, which I've been brought in connection with, like the work of Frederic Myers. He talks about the continuation of consciousness after death and actually did the rather classic experiment in which he communicated from the other side. There are books about this, recording this experiment, where he gave information to four different people, none of which made sense by itself. But when they put the pieces of it together, it was an intelligible communication. So that was an experiment from the other side that has become kind of a classic. Then there's all the work on spiritism. It's not proof, but there does seem to be something to it. Then there's the work on reincarnation, such as Ian Stevenson's research, work that's been done with people who report past-life experiences. There's a body of material that is developing that suggests there is some form of consciousness that is associated with a particular person that continues. I mean, we're not talking about the question, Is there consciousness in the universe? We're talking about a particular individual's consciousness continuing.

Then there's Gary Schwartz's controlled studies with mediums in which he shows that information was coming, that the mediums didn't know, and, apparently, could only have come from the relative on the other side. In other words, I can't say I know from my own experience, but I'm becoming familiar with literature from a number of different directions that supports this. But opinion is so a matter of opinion. It's in that area that has to do with experience as evidence, and we don't generally accept experience as evidence. Therefore this huge body of material tends to not be taken seriously, because it can't be proven in physicalistic or scientistic terms. But, evidently, it seems to be the case that there is some form of consciousness after the body dies. Then you have all of the spirit visitations from the so-called ghosts, some of which have been anchored in quite good research. So I don't know. I think the burden of proof has shifted in the direction of those who would deny it.

WHAT DO I THINK HAPPENS AFTER WE DIE?

I think about this question every day as an exercise of the imagination, and I frequently change my mind about it. Like Rupert Sheldrake, I suspect that what happens after we die is largely influenced by what we believe happens, much like in life.

Death is something that many people try to avoid thinking about, but I haven't been able to stop wondering about it since I was a child. One of the reasons I'm continually confronted with death is because I've been a longtime member of WAMM, which I discussed at the beginning of this chapter, and many of the members routinely exit this world. But it's much more than that. Our lives seem so fragile, the mysteries of birth and death surround us, and our time here is so short and precious.

Although I did have a mystifying experience that appeared to be genuine contact with someone after they died (which I will describe later in this chapter), and this did influence my perspective on death, I still entertain a new theory about what happens after we die almost every day, and I'm not even convinced that personal consciousness does survive death.

Nonetheless, here's one of my latest theories that I particularly like. It may be that our individual consciousness returns to its physical foundation after bodily death, the molecular awareness of the water, dirt, and condensed sunlight that literally composes our bodies and the biosphere, because I think that everything is conscious—all matter, energy, time, and space. Perhaps a condensation of our memories are preserved somehow in a type of postbiological field that we have yet to discover, or maybe not. But after we die I suspect that our primal sense of awareness may return to the original source of our consciousness—the ocean, the earth, and the sky. Of course, ultimately everything on Earth comes from the sun, so perhaps when we die we return to the solar goddess that spawned us and has always burned inside of us. Or maybe our souls are eaten by the moon, as the late Sufi mystic G. I. Gurdjieff claimed.

I suspect that all of our past thoughts remain forever etched into the space-time continuum, frozen like the frames of a motion picture, as our minds maintain the illusion of moving forward in time—although every thought that we've ever thought, every thought that we'll ever think, and every thought that we can possibly think, has and will always already exist in the Akashic Records. Either that or the hungry mischievous munchkins from the sixth dimension gobble up and eat our thoughts as we think them. I'm not sure.

MY NEAR-DEATH EXPERIENCE

After a woman whom I was deeply in love with broke up with me in 1995 I suffered from a case of severe depression. This eventually led to my psychotic episode with Zoloft, which I described earlier. The emotional pain was excruciating, and I continually contemplated suicide. In some desperate, crazed, and purely idiotic state, I called my ex-girlfriend and I told her that I was planning to kill myself. I was seriously considering doing it too. Two days later I was driving through the Santa Cruz Mountains, and as I was going around a sharp turn suddenly my steering column snapped and I couldn't control the direction of the car, which was headed right over a steep cliff. I experienced mind-screaming terror as time began moving in slow motion. I put the entire weight of my body on the brakes, but the car was moving too fast and I went flying straight off the cliff.

Once my car was in midair time completely stopped. I felt the presence of a higher intelligence with me, and the question being posed to me in this timeless moment was crystal clear: "You've been saying that you want to die, well here's your chance. Do you really want to die?" the disembodied voice asked. Thinking about all the people I loved, I knew in an instant that I wanted to live. I begged and pleaded for my life. Moments later the front of my car smashed into the side of the mountain around two hundred feet below. I was astonished to be alive. I looked up into the rearview mirror, expecting to see the worst, and didn't even see any blood. My car door was crunched in on the driver's side, so I had to climb out the passenger's side. Miraculously, I was able to climb up the mountain and call for help.

When the police arrived the officer told me that he had never seen anyone go over that cliff before and live, let alone walk away. I felt truly blessed and have never seriously considered suicide again. Life is simply too precious, and I now feel too strongly that I have an important mission to complete here.

When I interviewed psychologist Charles Tart, I asked him how a near-death experience (NDE) is similar to and different from a psychedelic experience. He replied:

> I wish that I could say we have a lot of studies that have made detailed phenomenological comparisons, but of course we haven't. The NDE is, of course, centered on the fact that you think that you've died, which is a pretty powerful centering device. It usually includes the feeling of moving through a tunnel, toward a light, contact with other beings, and a quick life review. A psychedelic experience may not have all of these characteristics. Some of the characteristics may be present, but certain details of the NDE may be missing, like the quick life review or the speedy return to normal consciousness. Now, this is interesting. This is one of the very vivid differences between psychedelic experiences and NDEs. With NDEs you can feel like you're way out there somewhere, and then "they" say that you have to go back, and bang! You're back in your body and everything is normal again. With psychedelics, of course, you come down more slowly and don't usually experience a condensed life review. . . . But psychedelic experiences also reach over a far wider terrain of possibilities.
>
> Let me tell you something about the life review. It's extremely common in NDEs for persons to undergo a life review, where they feel as if they remember at least every important event in their life, and often they say every single event in their life. Sometimes it even expands out into not only remembering and reliving every single event in their life but also into knowing psychically the reactions of other people to all their actions. For some it must be

horrible, because it seems that you would really experience their pain. I very seldom hear people say anything about a life review on psychedelics. Yeah, occasionally past memories have come up, but not this dramatic review of a person's whole life. There are sometimes consequences that overlap and are mutual, but I would say that the NDE is more powerful. It's more powerful in the sense that a person may make more drastic changes in their lifestyle or in their community if they try to integrate the acceptance of the NDE and make sense out of it. It's also more powerful in the sense that it's more liable to cause more lasting changes. A psychedelic experience can also have powerful life-changing effects. But let's face it: some people can pretty much forget their psychedelic experience afterward, much less alter their lives. It can simulate certain aspects of the NDE, but it doesn't carry the same force that the typical NDE does.

This actually rings true with my own experience. My psychedelic experiences were pale compared to the time that my car went over that cliff. For about a year afterward the experience allowed me to appreciate life in a completely new and joyous way, and it eliminated my fear of just about everything, including death. I felt so appreciative just to be alive, and the sight of sunlight twinkling through the leaves of a tree would bring tears of gratitude to my eyes. However, this new state of perception faded away after about a year, and I became my old neurotic self once again.

CONTACT WITH THE DEAD

My late friend Nina Graboi (whom I discussed in chapter 4 and interviewed for my book *Mavericks of the Mind*) and I often used to debate philosophical ideas pertaining to the mystery about what happens to consciousness after death. It was one of our favorite topics of conversation. In general, I took the position that after you die your individuality dissolves, and your sense of awareness merges with the universal one-ness, the source of everything, the mind of God.

On the other hand, Nina's position was, "Well, there is that, of course, but then there are all these levels in between, where individual-ity remains, besides the body, and you go through multiple incarnations with that." For years we went back and forth with these ideas. In our conversations Nina referred to her body as a *spacesuit*. She said that she was going to get a new spacesuit after she died, with memories from her previous lives carefully encoded, and that she would go from one space-suit to another each time she reincarnated.

After Nina died in 1999, late one night I was writing in my journal at a friend's house in Colorado and the TV was on, buzzing in the back-ground. I had eaten a cannabis cookie around an hour before and was thinking about what was going on in Nina's mind when she was dying. I thought to myself, *I'll bet Nina was thinking, "Now I see—David Jay Brown was right! You do just merge with the universal consciousness."* As I was sitting there reflecting on this, in a kind of egotistical, self-congratulatory way, I looked up and there on the television screen were just two words: SPACE SUIT.

A tingle traveled up my spine, I stopped writing in my journal, and my jaw dropped open. It was the most profound sense of com-munication with somebody after they died that I'd ever witnessed. That is the most compelling evidence I've personally experienced that consciousness not only continues after death but that some sense of individuality continues as well. Certainly other explanations could have accounted for this, but it was too striking to seem like just a mere coincidence. Still, I'm not entirely convinced. Maybe I just hal-lucinated it?

Regardless of what happens after we die, it's clear that cannabis and psychedelics can help to ease the suffering of people who are dying, and there is no reason why these substances shouldn't be avail-able to people who need them. It's bad enough that the authorities want to take away these sacred psychedelic plants from responsible adults here in America, the Land of the Free, but it's truly an outrage that they won't even allow the sick and dying to access them. Perhaps the reason why is because of this funny side effect that psychedelics have of causing people to question the assumptions of their culture, abandon consumerist lifestyles, and think differently. In the next chapter we'll be looking at how psychedelics have influenced every aspect of human culture, and how they are now revolutionizing the global mind and changing the world.

9
How Have Psychedelics Affected Human Culture?

Timothy Leary taught me that when influential people awaken to psychedelic awareness they are in a powerful position to really help change the world. This is why he and numerous others deliberately set out to try to expand the minds of talented artists, musicians, politicians, scientists, philanthropists, and religious leaders with psychedelics—and I think this noble endeavor to awaken this influential elite partially accounts for why our world has been changing so rapidly and dramatically over the past few decades.

Because psychedelics affect all aspects of the human mind, they affect every aspect of human culture. Science, art, medicine, politics, philosophy, and spirituality have all been transformed by individuals experienced with the psychedelic mind state, and the work that I have done with MAPS on their theme bulletins demonstrated how psychedelics have revolutionized the different frontiers of human culture.

To help understand the phenomena better, I asked many of the people I interviewed how psychedelics influenced their own work and their perspective on life. Some of the people were more comfortable talking about the benefits they gained from psychedelics than others, but I was persistent with those who were reluctant to speak about their use of psychedelics, as I considered it to be an important responsibility to record this influence for future generations.

Speaking out about one's personal use of psychedelic drugs is frightening for a lot of people as much of our present society has strong prejudices against them. I think the reluctance many people have about "coming out" about their use of psychedelics is similar to how many gay people have felt about publicly exposing their sexual orientation. (This is an important topic that my friend, University of Pennsylvania graduate student Nese Lisa Senol, has written about at length.) A number of people spoke to me publicly about their use of psychedelics for the first time, and more than a few of my interviewees spoke enthusiastically about how psychedelics had improved their lives, enhanced their creativity, and made them more spiritually aware.

SCIENCE AND PSYCHEDELICS

Each of the themes discussed in this chapter are, obviously, huge topics, deserving a whole encyclopedia devoted to them, so we'll just be able to get a few snapshots of this grand process here. A whole book could be written about science and psychedelics alone.

In the introduction to this book I discussed how the biotechnology revolution was largely started by two Nobel Prize–winning biochemists—Francis Crick and Kary Mullis—who both reportedly attributed part of their insights to their use of LSD. When I spoke with Mullis about how his use of psychedelics influenced his scientific work, as well as his perspective on life in general, he said:

> I would say that it was a mind-opening experience. It showed me that it might be a lot weirder here than I thought it was. So pay attention. Know what your assumptions are and which of those are just arbitrary. Notice that things might be a little bit different than you think they are. I wouldn't say that it led to any particular developments in my thought, except that it just expanded it a little bit.

I think almost anyone who's had those experiences would say that this place might be a little weirder than it appears. I'm not so certain anymore that the world is exactly the way I think it is. Most people get fairly stuck in ways of thinking that really are the current fashion, the current theory—like Newtonian mechanics seemed to be the way that things were for two hundred years.

Neuroscientist Candace Pert, who discovered the endorphin receptor in the brain, mentioned Aldous Huxley's classic book *The Doors of Perception* (about his experiences with mescaline) in her autobiographical book *Molecules of Emotion*. So I asked Pert if she ever had a psychedelic experience, and if so, how it had influenced her perspective on science and life. She replied:

I can say that I've had some unusual experiences. I basically missed the sixties, and even the seventies in terms of experimenting with drugs at the normal time, because I was a young mother and I was always in a very responsible authority-figure role from a very young age. But later on I experimented with marijuana and some of the psychedelics. I think the biggest influence was marijuana, which I didn't even try until I was, like, thirty-five years old. I think that had an impact on me, because it erases boundaries and gets you into interesting altered states. I've experimented with that, and less with some of the psychedelics. Has this influenced me? Sure. Spending time in an alternative reality, which is noncompetitive and loving, must have taken away my East Coast competitive nature. Of course, now I am convinced that marijuana should be avoided since it wreaks havoc with one's endocannabinoids.

Because Timothy Leary and Robert Anton Wilson suspected that cannabis and psychedelics are preparing us for life in the zero gravity of outer space, I was keen to speak with astronaut Edgar Mitchell about his consciousness-altering experience in outer space and how this experience might be similar to a psychedelic experience. I asked Mitchell if he ever had a psychedelic experience, and if so, how it compared with the mystical experience that he had while he was in space. Was there any similarity between these experiences? Mitchell replied:

> Yes, [I've had a psychedelic experience]. . . . It can [be similar to what I experienced in space]. What you're really doing here is opening channels in the brain to more perception. If you've studied any of Charlie Tart's work you know that there are many, many states of consciousness, and if you use psychedelics that is just a different state of consciousness. So what you're perceiving is different bits of information, and giving different meanings or attachments to it.

When I asked British biologist Rupert Sheldrake about how psychedelics have affected his perspective on science and life, he replied:

> I think that psychedelics reveal dimensions of the mind and experience that most of us would otherwise not experience. They show us there's a lot more going on than we're led to believe through textbooks on psychology and the standard kind of scientific model of the brain. I think they show that there are realms of experience that transcend ordinary waking consciousness, and for many people, including myself, I think psychedelics can reveal a world of consciousness and interconnection that is akin to mystical experience, of the kind experienced in many religious traditions. So I think in that sense the psychedelic experience is akin to mysticism, indeed is a kind of mysticism. And by *mysticism* I don't mean "obscurantism." I mean "direct conscious experience of expanded realms of consciousness or other regions of consciousness, which go beyond those we normally experience in our everyday lives."

Lucid dream researcher Stephan LaBerge also spoke with me about psychedelics. When I asked him if his experience with psychedelics influenced his research, he replied:

> In a way. It was one of the things that inspired me to take an interest in the mind and before that . . . I had no interest in the mind; I was interested only in the outside world. At first I wanted to be making analogs of tryptamines, because I was thinking we just need to modify these molecules and then they'll really work, instead of almost telling you all. That was my naïveté, not realizing that the problem wasn't the molecule, the problem was the mind. From going from the ordinary state of perceiving the world to an extraordinary state of perceiving the world, I would think, *So this is what it's really like!* Of course, the next day when I was back in the usual state, comparing the two, I realized, of course, that wasn't what it was like and this is not what it's like. They're both mental models or simulations. It's something that was very important for me, in terms of understanding the power of the mind, and seeing how just changing some of the operational parameters in the perceptual system could lead to a radically different view of the world. I think it's shocking and a tragedy what's happened with the illegality of these substances, preventing scientific research and therapeutic use, and I look forward to the day when that changes.

I spoke with the late psychiatric researcher John Mack about psychedelics as well. I asked him if he ever had a psychedelic experience, and if so, how it influenced his perspective on science and life. He replied:

> Yeah, I've had psychedelic experiences, as have many people who don't necessarily want to talk about it. What psychedelic experiences do is remove the veil. They remove the barrier between yourself and the surround, so that you experience a much more powerful

vibrational connection with the world around you. You experience something like, I guess, what people call the divine, or a basic creative force. It opens you to that. Many people who have moved into what is called the new paradigm, or the new worldview, have, at some point, been jump-started by psychedelic experiences. I mean, you could do a study of that if you wanted. I think the resistance to psychedelics in the culture is not because they're medically threatening so much—I guess people could have bad trips—but because, by taking away the veil of socialization that lies on top of our true selves, people then become openhearted, open-minded, think for themselves, and are less likely to be programmable by the conventional media or the socioeconomic system we live in. It isn't like a conspiracy, but there's an intuition in the established collective that psychedelics are threatening to it, because, as I say, people who have opened their hearts, minds, and souls through that means—or any other means that undoes the programming that we've all taken in—begin to question, think for themselves, don't accept the political lies or the inequalities that exist. Or they feel more connected with the environment, so they find viscerally abhorrent the whole deterioration of the environment and the commercial callousness that is at the root of that. So I think they're very threatening. I don't work in this area, but I'm interested in the resistance to psychedelics as a cultural or political phenomenon. And, at this point, I'm persuaded of their power.

Physicist and author Peter Russell also shared his perspective on psychedelics with me. I asked him if he ever had a psychedelic experience, and if so, how it influenced his perspective on science and spirituality. He replied:

Yes, although I don't think it influenced my perspective on science greatly. I see science as a valid way of exploring the nature of the material world and arriving at consensus truth about this world. The problem with science is that it assumes this material reality is the only reality. I was aware of these limitations to science before I had a psychedelic experience. Having that sort of experience just confirmed my understanding that science was a partial perspective on the cosmos—valid within its own frame of reference, but only partial. What changed was my appreciation of the spiritual. I realized there was validity to a lot of what the great spiritual teachers, saints, and mystics had spoken about. And I realized there were other ways of construing reality, other ways of creating one's own experience. But the most important part of the psychedelic experience was that, at times, I could let go completely of the ego mode and be with an experience without the illusion of the ego—of me here experiencing something. I could touch into that sense of oneness that the mystics have spoken about. It was many years ago, back in the sixties when I did this. And, for me, it was a factor in my saying that I need to look at Eastern mysticism much more deeply. Because I think, like many people back then who tried these substances, it led to a different appreciation of reality, a whole opening up to a new way of seeing things, and a new understanding of spirituality. However, the next day you're back with memories, or maybe some shift in experience, but over time it fades. I realized that yogis, monks, and others in the East had been exploring the mind, in natural ways, for thousands of years and came up with a wealth of wisdom about how to tap in to these deeper states of consciousness. They learned how to dissolve this sense of ego through natural means, such as meditation and other such practices. So you could say that the psychedelic experience spurred me to find ways of raising consciousness that didn't involve psychedelics. And that's really been my mission in life: to draw upon what these inner seekers and explorers have found and to try to integrate this into my own life and pass it on to others, because that is the most important need in the world today.

John Polk Allen was the driving force behind the development of the Biosphere 2 project in the Arizona desert. Biosphere 2 is the largest self-sustaining ecosystem ever built, a masterpiece of human engineering. Inside the sealed 3.15-acre biosphere are miniature replicas of all the Earth's environments, designed to function together as a single system. The relevance of Biosphere 2 lies in the light it sheds on our understanding of the Earth's biosphere and its value as a prototype for permanent life habitats on suitable locations in space. I asked Allen if psychedelics had influenced his work on this project. He replied:

> The Biosphere 2 couldn't have been built without the help of a number of shamans who are probably the primary ethnobotanists in the world. It's impossible to fully appreciate the Amazon or anything as complex as a tropical rain forest without special states of consciousness. What's used in the Amazon by the shaman are substances such as *Banisteriopsis caapi* and beta harmaline. These substances put people in a state where they can see eidetically instead of just sensationally. The forests and this eidetic ability is what makes the shaman an essential partner of all ethnobotanists. The people who painted the Lascaux caves were eidetic—that is, they must have seen the animal so clearly that they could copy the eidetic image, and nobody could paint like that until the Renaissance. Without this eidetics of sensation and memory, which are successionally linked, you can't, in my opinion, comprehend a complex totality. Eidetics are so unknown to people in the modern world, and without that kind of vision I doubt that total systems will spread very far, because people just won't see it. Our senses are reductionist. If you go by memory then we're remembering only our successive sensations or we're combining them by an active imagination which produces an element of fantasy. But if we've had an eidetic image, then we can have a memory that, when we train it, can then reproduce that image, but it's possible to have an eidetic experience without being

able to remember it. Coca chewing is quite legal in South America and is used for endurance. If you're doing major studies in the mountains or in the forest with the Indians, then you need to use it to keep up with them. I've also participated in shamanic ceremonies because I think that it's important to see the total system in a very literal sense.

I asked revolutionary mathematician Ralph Abraham if his experiences with psychedelics had any influence on his mathematical perspective and work. He replied:

Yes. I guess my experiences with psychedelics influenced everything. . . . There was a period of six or seven years that included psychedelics, traveling in Europe, sleeping in the street, my travels in India, living in a cave, and so on. These were all part of the walkabout between my first mathematical period and all that has followed in the past fifteen years. This was my hippie period, this spectacular experience of the gylanic revival . . . of the sixties. I think my emphasis on vibrations and resonance is one thing that changed after my walkabout. Another thing that changed, which had more to do with psychedelics than with India, was that I became more concerned with the application of mathematics to the important problems of the human world. I felt, and continue to feel, that this planet is really sick. There are serious problems that need to be faced, and if mathematics doesn't have anything to do with these problems, then perhaps it isn't worth doing. One should do something else. So I thought vigorously after that period about something I had not even thought about before: the relationship of the research to the problems of the world. That became an obsession, I would say.

PSYCHEDELICS AND POPULAR CULTURE

How do television, video games, and popular culture affect us? The answer appears to be "a lot." When speaking to an audience of ravers, British comedian Marcus Alexander Brigstocke is noted for having said, "If Pac-Man had affected us as kids, we'd all be running around in dark rooms, munching magic pills, and listening to repetitive electronic music."

Numerous references to psychedelic drugs—as well as the influence of psychedelic mind states—can be clearly and pervasively seen throughout popular culture. If you know where to look, psychedelic influences and references appear just about everywhere—in film, music, television, comedy, advertising, comic books, fashion, toys, video games, and other multimedia art forms. Sometimes the reference or influence is blatantly obvious, while other times it is subtle, or hidden with a knowing wink. This is especially true with regard to youth culture.

Douglas Rushkoff is a media theorist and one of the world's experts on youth culture. When Rushkoff's first book on media theory, *Media Virus!,* was published in 1994, some critics initially viewed his upbeat assessments of how teenagers were playfully deconstructing mass media as too idealistic. His idea, which quickly became popular with younger generations, went against the conventional assumption that computer games and MTV videos were necessarily bad for kids. Rushkoff contended that the new interactive information technologies had the power to accelerate thought and increase intelligence.

Rushkoff's enthusiasm for youth culture and new technology seemed reminiscent of Timothy Leary's optimism, and, in fact, Rushkoff's theories about media built on Leary's idea that each generation is a new breed of human—almost a new species—and that kids nowadays have nervous systems that process information in ways that are faster and less linear than previous generations. Rushkoff also expanded on British biologist Richard Dawkins's concept of memes—units of culture that replicate like genes—to create a "media virus," an idea that spreads through populations via the media.

Ironically, after mainstream businesses and respected academics started to take Rushkoff's ideas and observations about media and youth culture seriously (simply because his theories had true predictive value), some people in the digital counterculture saw Rushkoff as something of a sellout, largely because he began consulting for Fortune 500 companies. But Rushkoff defended his actions by saying that he has always stayed true to his ideals. Whether he's addressing a corporate-culture or a counterculture audience, Rushkoff has always aimed to be a cheerleader for change, growth, cooperation, and creativity—what Timothy Leary would have called an evolutionary agent. He is trying to help the human race evolve, and one of the ways to do that, he believes, is to break down the artificial distinction between "us" and "them."

When I spoke with Rushkoff, I asked him how his experience with psychedelics influenced his writing and his perspective on life. He replied:

I think it's very hard for anyone who has had psychedelic experiences to ever know how many of the insights that they might credit to psychedelia might have happened anyway. In other words, sometimes I think, *Okay, it's all the acid.* That you have one acid trip and, basically, you never come down from it—just the rest of life kind of comes up to it. That there's a full categorical shift in the way you understand the world, that your perspective is forever changed, and that's it. But I talk to a lot of people who've never had psychedelic experiences—at least chemical- or plant-induced ones, or who have never even smoked pot—and they still seem just as aware of the fact that we're all living in reality tunnels and that we chose different tunnels. And they can have moments of a broader perspective where they see the way all these things are arbitrarily chosen, and that we've been living in a certain picture frame, and how you can pull out of that frame and see all these other possibilities. So the only thing I know for sure is that psychedelics provide a very tangible and experiential metaphor for the interchangeable contextual frames that we use to understand the world we live in. For me, certainly, psychedelics were a valuable medicine—for a kid who, at nineteen, was really trapped in doing premed and becoming a doctor. I was going to do all this stuff I didn't really want to do. I actually made the decision to go be a theater person before I'd had any kind of drug experience, but it definitely helped. Afterward it helped me see the validity of that decision, and it helped me understand that all this recontextualizing I had been doing, all of the frames within frames. All of the theater that I was so interested in was not for the play but for the proscenium arch itself and for the ritual that was going on in the room. All of that had a shamanic history, and it was a bit more universally applicable than I had realized. It wasn't just something that happened in a theater; it's something that happens in the world at every moment. We are contextualizing and recontextualizing things based on assumptions.

When I asked Robert Anton Wilson how his use of psychedelics influenced his writings and his view of the world, he replied:

I've moved from atheism to agnosticism, with somewhat pantheistic leanings. I just don't want to sound too pretentious about it. I don't claim to know anything about any gods or goddesses, but I suspect a good deal. I suspect that some form of divinity probably exists, but it seems to me immanent and decentralized, not transcendent and authoritarian. More like Internet than like a monarchy. Aleister Crowley said, "Every man and every woman is a star." We in the Guns and Dope Party have changed that to "Every man and every woman is a tsar." That not only signifies scientific and political freedom but also something in the neighborhood of Vedic identification of the true self with divinity, or at least the Quaker inner light.

I asked the late comedian George Carlin how marijuana and his use of psychedelics affected his comedy career and his perspective on life. He replied:

What they did was affect my consciousness, obviously, and that affects everything about you. So, naturally, in this line of work it's extremely important, extremely influential. Your consciousness influences the work. I was an early pot smoker. I was smoking pot when I was thirteen in 1950. It was an unheard of act in an Irish American neighborhood. People didn't know anything about it and considered it to be on a level with heroin. I mean, it was just . . . [speaks in a scratchy old-geezer voice] marijuana—you smoke one of those things, and yeah, boy, you're gone for life. So we were kind of a daring little group of us. We were on a new generational cusp. . . .

I think that marijuana is a consciousness-altering drug that has a cumulative effect. I also think it is a self-limiting drug, if a person is paying attention. It is a drug that suggests its own disuse, eventually. Some people maintain a certain consumption, at a good level, and they're not just half-asleep all the time and can't think. They save it for nighttime, or the weekend, or whatever, and that's different. But generally marijuana and LSD . . . they're certainly not in the narcotic classes, stimulants, or any of those things. They are separate. LSD—originally as unaltered by man—along with peyote, pot, and those forms of hallucinogens, are all completely natural. They come from nature, and the only things that are done with them is they're passed from one person to another. It's these other drugs—where we get in the laboratory or the garage and we start altering their molecular structure—that are the deadly ones. The really deadly things have come from man's altering of nature, of the parts he can manipulate.

Pot is an herb. It's very natural. It obviously has some healing qualities and some palliative qualities. I think it changed my thinking. It fostered offbeat thinking, the kind of alternative thinking that was already an internal part of me—this disbelief in the received wisdom and in the authority, as it was passed along. I think it fostered that. Then it changed my comedy. I was a straight, mainstream, suit-and-tie comic for ten years, from 1960 to 1969 or '70. I had a two-tiered life going on, and I didn't even know it. One of them was this law-breaking, school-quitting, pot-smoking person, with no respect for authority. The other one was a mainstream dream. I wanted to be in the movies. I wanted to be Danny Kaye. Well, you can't be Danny Kaye if you're going to be this other thing. So I lived two lives. My professional life was this straight path of pleasing the public.

It wasn't until the late sixties that things changed, and this was because of the alternative culture—the people I could really identify with, what's called the counterculture. This began to manifest itself through the youth culture, with its disrespect for authority, free love, and "Let's get high," and "Here's how I feel," and "Here's what's going on in my mind and my heart." All those things had been suppressed in America—some voluntarily, some not—prior to that. The fifties are notorious for that. But jazz and the beatniks were the exception. The bohemian world. But they were just starting.

Anyway, I was attracted to this other thing in the late sixties, because all my friends were musicians who had gone through the changes already. I was a big pot smoker. But slowly I used a little peyote, a little mescaline, and these tendencies in me to be myself and not play a fake role as a people-pleasing, mainstream comedian came to the fore. I became more myself. The comedy became more personal, therefore more political and therefore more successful. I think you can never be successful unless you are yourself, at least certainly not successful in the good, rich sense of the word. So, suddenly, I also became materially successful. People started buying albums. I had four Gold albums in a row. So the LSD, directly—in conjunction with its role in the counterculture, and my taking of it, those two things—definitely changed my life, because my creativity shifted into a very high gear.

Comedian and yippie movement cofounder Paul Krassner told me about how his experience with psychedelics influenced his satirical writings, his comedy, and his perspective on life. He said:

> On some levels it's impossible to know. There are concepts that I probably wouldn't have gotten without them—like saying that what really gets you high is the glue that's on the rolling paper, not the pot inside the joint. I don't think I would have come up with that concept, among many others, if I hadn't been high. I wouldn't have a lot of the stuff I've done on stage, which is just talking about experiences like taking acid at the Chicago Conspiracy Trial. Obviously I couldn't write about those things or talk about them if I hadn't done them. It would never have occurred to me to have those kind of stories. But also it's the process. I mean, sometimes it's impossible to know. If an idea comes to me and I'm stoned, how do I know whether I would have gotten that same idea if I were not stoned? Or vice versa even? So I just surrender to the process. But I know that being stoned seems to help me make connections and to extrapolate on notions. There's a lot of comics who get ideas when they're stoned and will then put those ideas into the material when they write something. Whereas, say, George Carlin has said that he will work on, work on, work on something, and then smoke some pot to help him fine-tune it. Then there are people who will perform when they're stoned. So there's all different levels of the relationship.

When I asked the late beat poet Allen Ginsberg about how his experiences with psychedelics affected his writing and life in general, he said:

> I wrote a couple of good poems on them—with mescaline, acid, nitrous oxide, marijuana, and amphetamines. So those are direct influences on my writing. But aside from sixty or so pages, the spiritual effect of drugs was not extensive in creation of texts.

Celebrated magician Jeff McBride also spoke with me about psychedelics. I asked him if he ever had a psychedelic experience, and if so, how it affected his perspective on magic. He replied:

The answer to that is yes. What I've learned is that . . . let me think about this for a second. It has changed the way I do, where I choose to do it, and how much I do. Set and setting and dosage. In Las Vegas the setting is a casino. The mind-set is, "Let's see how good this guy is." Or "Let's go kill an hour before we lose our wallets at the gaming tables, right?" And the dosage is, you have to hit these people over the head. They're pretty jaded, because in Las Vegas they have to walk down the street, past exploding volcanos and giant water fountains. So to even reach their aesthetic awareness you have to kind of bombard them with images and visuals. . . . The way I do this is by meeting that demand at the top of my show. Then I put on the brakes and go into complete stillness and silence, challenging that in a conventional theater setting. I do things in my Las Vegas show that no magician has ever attempted. Total silence. No music. No movement. No action on stage for four minutes, and see if I can totally entrance the audience. And I have stunning results with it—because they are expecting one thing, and as soon as I deliver the expectation, I can take them into new territory, which is stillness.

To self-publish your own books and have them wind up on the *New York Times* bestseller list is an almost unheard of phenomenon, yet Peter McWilliams did it six times. Peter had a gift for writing about universal themes—such as love and loss—with great clarity and simplicity, in a way that many people can relate to. His work has inspired millions of people, and his books have personally helped me through some of the most difficult times in my life. In his lifetime he wrote and published more than thirty books, including *Do It!, Life 101, Wealth 101, You Can't Afford the Luxury of a Negative Thought,* and *How to Survive the*

Loss of a Love. I asked Peter how psychedelics influenced his work or his perspective on life. He replied:

> By the time of 1969, when I started transcendental meditation, I had taken acid several times. I was an agnostic. I mean, it's hard to come out of an LSD experience and still believe there's an external God. . . . God is in everything, including us. That is what you find on LSD, and that is exactly what Jesus said: "The kingdom of Heaven is within you. . . . Our Father who art in Heaven." That's two direct quotes from Jesus. One of the least quoted of all of the direct quotes of Jesus. The Pharisees asked him, "Where is the kingdom of Heaven?" "The kingdom of Heaven," he said, "is within you." Then when his disciples said, "Teach us how to pray," the first line was, "Our Father, who art in Heaven." Where's Heaven? Within you. . . . Jesus said, "To enter the kingdom of Heaven you must become like a child." And what's a child like? What does marijuana do but turn you into a child? It turns you into a curious, delightful, living-in-the-moment, sensual being.

Reverend Ivan Stang, the leading force behind the Church of the SubGenius—a brilliant and hilarious satirical spoof of organized religion—spoke with me about the relationship between the church and psychedelics. Many people who use psychedelics are big fans of the church, and their prophet—J. R. "Bob" Dobbs—has appeared on sheets of blotter acid. I asked Stang about this connection. He said:

> Well, I wish I could explain that. For some reason this whole thing seems to attract potheads like crazy. Now, of course, I haven't met every one of these ten thousand people I'm talking about, but I've met a hell of a lot of them. And from what I can tell, about 85 percent of them are probably some kind of psychedelic drug user. Now, why that is, you got me. There's nothing terribly overt about that in any of the books. In fact, it actually says that with Bob, you can

throw away all your cheap conspiracy street drugs and never come down.

I asked Stang what role psychedelics played in the development of the Church of the SubGenius and in his personal development. He replied:

It's hard to put one's finger on that exactly. I mean, somehow I can imagine it all happening just fine without a lot of psychedelics involved. Personally, speaking for myself, I actually did write a whole lot of that first book, and I was a very well-behaved boy at that time. I wasn't really touching anything except, well, about halfway through. I'd had a terrible freak-out on LSD when I was sixteen years old. It almost killed me. And when I was sixteen I had not even tried beer. I was very leery of alcohol, and I had not even been drunk. I had been stoned on pot I think a couple of times before I took my first hit of LSD in 1969. All my high school buddies were doing it. They could drop acid and go to football practice or take exams. Well, it didn't really agree with me. I was a very insecure kid, and it was a very close call. If it hadn't been for that nervous breakdown caused by LSD, and my own insecurity, and a bunch of fucking Jack Webb antidrug propaganda that helped fuel the panic of it all, I probably would just be a nameless special-effects technician doing detailing on miniatures in Hollywood—which is not bad. But when I had this terrible freak-out as a very young man, I didn't want my parents to know this had happened, and I had to deal with it in my own way. My interests changed quite a bit after that. My entire approach to life completely changed. I was sort of schizoid, paranoid, and terrified after that trip; for a while. I thought that I would never be able to experience fun or slack or any kind of relaxation again. I thought I would always be on my guard against flashbacks for the rest of my life. I had two choices: I could either kill myself, or I could forget myself and remember that everybody else around me still had the capability of having fun, happiness, and enjoying, and that I could help them do that. As corny as this sounds, at the age of seventeen, thanks to a bad drug trip, I actually decided that maybe I better devote myself to serving others rather than myself. That all sounds real good, and I surely lapsed back into normal self-ishness several months later, when I discovered that alcohol was the perfect cure for LSD psychosis. Unfortunately, several years later, of course, I had to quit drinking alcohol, and by then I'd forgotten about being such a nice guy. But for a while there I might as well have been like a wonderful little Catholic Jesuit monk, dedicated to the service of others.

ART AND PSYCHEDELICS

Among the many astonishing things that psychedelic substances do to the human nervous system, they have a most extraordinary effect on visual perception, the imagination, and the optical cortex of the brain.

Visual art that is reminiscent of the kinds of perceptual changes that psychedelics bestow on our view of the world and the extraordinary visions that one sees with closed eyes during a psychedelic brain state—ever-morphing, intricately detailed, brightly colored, otherworldly, complex, geometrically organized, and imbued with personal meaning—is often referred to as psychedelic or visionary art.

Psychedelic art is not always inspired by a drug-induced experience, but it often is, and like dreams and surreal art, visionary artists draw on the unconscious as their source of inspiration. However, truly psychedelic paintings are charged with an unmistakable psychoactive intensity that clearly demonstrates that the artist has intimate knowledge of profound mystical states of consciousness.

Sex, death, and spiritual transcendence are common commingling themes in psychedelic art, and this type of art is, of course, usually best viewed and most appreciated while one is under the influence of a psychedelic. Most people who have done psychedelics can instantly tell if a piece of artwork was inspired by a psychedelic experience or not, as knowledge of psychedelic mind states simply cannot be faked.

Artists, musicians, and other creative people seem to take naturally to the psychedelic experience, and scientific studies by the late psychiatric researcher Oscar Janiger demonstrated that LSD can enhance the creative performance of artists. This doesn't mean that LSD will necessarily make one more creative; rather, it means that if one already has a creative talent, then LSD has the potential to amplify this.

Psychedelic art is certainly nothing new. It's been around for as long as human beings have been eating strange plants and painting on cave walls. Currently there are so many new and talented psychedelic artists emerging on the art scene that it's hard to keep up.

One of my favorite psychedelic artists is painter Alex Grey. Grey's work often depicts naked translucent people, as though they were caught in the midst of a mystical experience, with uncanny scientific precision. Grey's paintings are painstakingly detailed, revealing anatomically accurate views of the inner body. Intricate blood-vascular configurations, eerie skeletal structures, and nervous systems that are exploding with electrical activity are visible inside bodies that radiate spiritual auras, acupuncture meridians, and metaphysical energies.

The subjects are often engaged in activities that make the most of this incredible, eyeball-grabbing technique that "X-rays" multiple levels of reality simultaneously. Grey applies this multidimensional perspective to such archetypal human experiences as being born, dying, praying, meditating, and making love. I find that merely looking at one of his paintings can trigger a mystical state of consciousness. Grey did the cover of my second book of interviews, *Voices from the Edge,* and I interviewed him for my book *Conversations on the Edge of the Apocalypse.* When I spoke with Grey about how psychedelics have affected his life and work, he said:

When I came back from the North Magnetic Pole, I knew I was looking for something. I was twenty-one, and I was searching for

God. I didn't know what that was. I was an existentialist. Within twenty-four hours of returning from the pole I was invited to a party by an acquaintance who would become my wife. She invited me along with our professor, so the professor took me there. On the way he offered me a bottle of Kahlúa laced with a high dose of LSD. It was the end of school, and I decided to celebrate. I drank a good deal of it. Allyson drank the rest. That was my first LSD experience. Tripping that night I experienced going through a spiritual rebirth canal inside of my head. I was in the dark, going toward the light, spinning in this tunnel, a kind of an opalescent living mother-of-pearl tube. All paradoxes were resolved in this tunnel—dark and light, male and female, life and death. It was a very strong archetypal experience. The next day, because it had been my first trip, I called Allyson up to talk to her about it. I asked her out that night, and we never left each other. It's been over twenty years. Within twenty-four hours of announcing that I'm looking for God, an LSD experience opened me up on a spiritual, evolutionary path, and I had met my wife. It was miraculous. My prayers were answered. Allyson and I have maintained an ongoing psychedelic sacramental relationship. We have often tripped laying in bed, blindfolded, or in a beautiful environment. Then, coming out of blindfolds, we write and draw.

I asked Grey if he ever tried to do any painting while he was tripping. He replied:

A little—the results are interesting and remind me of the trip, but it's not my most successful work. My work takes a steady mind, eye, and hand to accomplish. The psychedelic helps me to access the infinitude of the imagination, allowing me to see countless interpenetrating dimensions. William James says that no model of reality can be complete without taking these alternative dimensions of consciousness into account. Since I want to make art dealing with the nature of consciousness and spirit, I have to experience higher dimensions of consciousness. During a trip I will have visions that are crystallizations of my life experience, or something completely surprising. You may enter a dimension that you've never known before, and it seems very real, more real than this phenomenal world. That other reality seems to be tinkering with this one, or acting like a puppet master to this one. I want to reveal the interrelationships between the different dimensions in my work. . . . Making interdimensionality visible validates it for people who have had that experience. They can see a picture outside of their own heads and say, "It was something like this. I'm not crazy." There's plenty of people who've had those experiences. Perhaps the work can be useful in that way. I've talked to people who use my paintings as a tool to access the dimensions that are represented. Some people trip and look at the book, or look at the art, and key into the states that are symbolized there. That is a psychedelic or entheogenic full circle. I glimpsed the visions while tripping, came back, and made the work. Then people trip and access the higher state that produced the vision. The painting acts a portal to the mystical dimension. That is the real usefulness of the work, and it is the great thing about any sacred art.

Another personal favorite is Big Sur painter and poet Carolyn Mary Kleefeld, whom I discussed earlier. Kleefeld juxtaposes ecstatic visions with the beauty of the natural world on canvas, and there is a profoundly joyous quality to her abstract expressionistic work. Her pieces seem like picture postcards from the highest heavens. Kleefeld paints portals into a higher-dimensional world that blends the organic fluidity of life with transcendent mystical qualities, alchemically weaving together an enchanted paradisical landscape that is inhabited by timeless mythic archetypes, unique biological forms and strange creatures, giggling nature spirits, and radiant explosions of erotic energy.

Computer graphic animator Brummbaer stylishly blends mathematical precision with sensuous human sexuality and fabricates fantastic polymorphic worlds that look like photographs of ayahuasca visions. His animated alien worlds are composed of fractal-organized interlocking tubular networks and spinning hyperdimensional objects encoded with cryptic esoteric messages. Brummbaer says that his philosophy of creativity stems from his notion that an artist is but "a humble window washer." His computer screen is simply a window, he says, that allows us to see through into other worlds, and all he does is polish the screen so that we can see through them to the other side.

I asked Brummbaer what role psychedelics played in influencing his artwork. He replied:

> A profoundly trivial influence. You close your eyes when you're tripping, and you wish everybody could see what you're seeing. You wish there was a way to get it out of your mind, objectify it, and make it visible to other people. Ever since computers came around we are getting closer to being able to reproduce these psychedelic visions.

Swiss artist H. R. Giger is another personal favorite. Giger is perhaps best known for designing (and winning an Academy Award for) the creatures and sets in the original science-fiction horror film *Alien,* although his paintings, which have appeared popularly as posters and on record album covers, are actually even more extraordinary. Giger is the master of capturing the bad trip. If one were able to freeze a moment from Edgar Allen Poe or H. P. Lovecraft's worst psychedelic nightmares, we would probably have an image that very much resembled one of Giger's pieces.

Macabre metallic biomechanical creatures erotically slither through his dark, decaying landscapes, locked in a gruesome orgy of repulsive torment, while dirty gray cyborgs grind together over carpets of screaming mutilated baby heads. When I interviewed Giger, he said that he has always been fascinated by the combination of "elegance and horror" and that some of his pieces were inspired by LSD experiences. His work provides us with a tour through the interior chambers of Hell, the darkest regions of our souls, and it is certainly not for the squeamish. But to some it can be so horrific that it becomes extremely beautiful.

Celebrated artist Robert Williams, whose early work with *Zap Comix* is among some of my very favorite comic art, has also been outspoken about how psychedelics have affected his work. He said:

> They influenced it tremendously. . . . My work before psychedelics was kind of like a Wallace Wood style . . . he was big influence on me too. It was kind of like a street element, hot-rod Wallace Wood effect I had in my work. Maybe a little science-fiction fantasy. But when psychedelics came along, it opened up the world of color and shape; an emphasis was put on things that were really not paid attention to before. The predominant thing about psychedelics is harsh contrast, working one color against another. That had been done by the German Expressionists, but it wasn't done like this. The German Expressionists like to get one color against another color to make it ugly—real dark green against harsh pink, for example—and it would be this real obtrusive thing. But psychedelic art wasn't like that; it was colors at their maximum. It's like a hundred percent yellow against a hundred percent red. . . . It's like putting green up against a red-orange, so where they touched each other your eye would vibrate. Then op art came along, which was a product of psychedelic art. That had like a two or three year hiatus, and then fell out.

> When I was working for Roth, I had to render a lot of automobile stuff. He always hired a lot of artists that were technical illustrators to do really slick automotive renderings. There was a fellow there named Ed Newton who could do the best chrome in the world. The smooth chrome would just make your mouth water, but his imagination wouldn't let him take it any further than car or industrial surfaces. He showed me the formulas for working chrome. So, being psychedelic, man, I just saw all the possibilities to that shit on water, air, women—everything. So that chrome center spread that you're talking about was my first attempt to make everything chrome

in the picture. In fact, that's a reproduction of it on a mirror up there. A fellow from England sent that to me. That's the Rosetta Stone of chrome there. It tells you how to handle any shape. So I'm talking about '67, '68. I started doing this, and it got out in the car magazines, and before long, advertising agencies started picking up on this. I started having advertising agencies calling me. J. Walter Thompson called me, but I couldn't get along with them, and I didn't want to be bossed by them. Inside three or four years the entire advertising thing—all over the United States, Europe, and the world—started having chrome lettering. The chrome lettering you see today started with me. So I netted exactly nothing out of that. There were a number of artists who made pretty good livings off doing chrome. . . . When I got into it, I got really deep into it. I started figuring, *Well this is a stylization, and I've got a language going with a whole new form of visual surface control. And if I get deeper into this, I'm going to find something even better.* I started getting more abstract, and getting deeper into working with this. . . . Instead of making it look like chrome, I started changing the colors on it, trying to alter the language, so it doesn't read properly as chrome, yet the language is there. It's psychedelic as hell. It's obvious that the guy who did this has taken some drugs.

MUSIC AND PSYCHEDELICS

Probably the first artistic medium that springs to mind when most people think of psychedelics is music. From the Grateful Dead, to Jimi Hendrix, Jefferson Airplane, the Beatles, Ozric Tentacles, Smashing Pumpkins, Infected Mushroom, and Shpongle, an endless array of talented musicians have claimed inspiration from psychedelics, and a sizable percentage of the audiences at many large, outdoor music festivals are often high on cannabis or tripping on psychedelics.

Music is often an integral part of many people's psychedelic experiences, and it is even used in many clinical, therapeutic settings with psychedelics. It appears that this tradition of combining music and psychedelics stretches back into human prehistory, as some members of our species have been tripping on psychedelic plants and dancing to music at nightlong ceremonies and festivals since the beginning of time.

One of the many delightful things that people often say that they enjoy about listening to music—with the enhancement of a psychedelic drug or plant—is how they can see exquisitely patterned, closed-eye visual patterns and bright colors that dance and move to the music, in corresponding rhythms and beats, as a synesthetic blurring of the senses is commonly reported.

There is probably no band of musicians more lovingly associated with the use of psychedelics than the Grateful Dead. I spoke with the late lead guitarist for the band, Jerry Garcia, and when I asked him how psychedelics had influenced his music, he said:

> Phew! I can't answer that. There was a me before psychedelics and a me after psychedelics. That's the best I can say. I can't say that it affected the music specifically; it affected the whole me. The problem of playing music is essentially of muscular development, and that is something you have to put in the hours to achieve no matter what. There isn't something that strikes you and suddenly you can play music. . . . I think that psychedelics was part of music for me in so far as I'm a person who was looking for something and psychedelics and music are both part of what I was looking for. They fit together, although one didn't cause the other.

Arguably, not since the Grateful Dead has a brand of popular music been so lovingly associated with psychedelics as the electronica music project known as Shpongle. Psychedelics have played a huge role in the creation, performance, and experience of Shpongle's music, which is extremely popular among members of the psychedelic community. I interviewed British electronic musician Simon Posford (a.k.a., Hallucinogen), who, along with Australian musician Raja Ram, created

Shpongle. Posford is generally responsible for coordinating the synthesizers, studio work, and live instrumentation, while Ram contributes broad musical concepts, inspiration, and flute arrangements. I spoke with Posford about how psychedelics have influenced his experience with music, and I asked him how it has affected his creativity and his performance. He replied:

> I would say massively, and on a profound level. In fact, so fundamentally that I didn't even really like the type of music that I now create before I took psychedelics. I liked bands and music with singers and stuff. I never got into Kraftwerk or Depeche Mode or any of the well-known electronic bands that my friends would listen to. Then, once I took psychedelics, I really went off that for a while, and only wanted to hear the alien, otherworldly, futuristic sounds of electronic music, and it's what inspired me to start making the music that I'm doing now. In a way it's foundational to what I'm doing, because it pushed me down this path. Also, it changed my appreciation of music in general. I think that listening to music in an altered state of consciousness can either magnify the music or it can really leave you cold. Hopefully it will enrich the experience, and hence we have what we call psychedelic music, which is designed to do so. I think that electronic music can certainly enhance a psychedelic experience. I probably shouldn't mention the artist, but there's a particularly commercial band who sold a lot of records in the eighties and early nineties, and I made the terrible mistake of listening to their music while trying to have a psychedelic experience in my parents' house when I was a teenager. I put on this CD while I was tripping and truly heard it for the bland potbellied corporate, insipid, vapid nastiness that it was. So our only concerns now are, What do we need to do to make this sort of kaleidoscopic music that really expands the brain in the same way that, I think, psychedelics do?

MEDICINE AND PSYCHEDELICS

MAPS, the Beckley Foundation, the Council on Spiritual Practices, and the Heffter Research Institute are all currently supporting research with psychedelics as treatments for a variety of medical disorders—from alcoholism and drug addiction to post-traumatic stress disorder and cluster headaches—with great success. I suspect that it won't be long before psychedelic drugs are recognized as legitimate medical tools.

Andrew Weil, M.D., whom we discussed in chapter 5, is an internationally recognized expert on integrative medicine, which combines the best therapies of conventional and alternative medicine. Dr. Weil's lifelong study of medicinal herbs, mind-body interactions, and alternative medicine has made him one of the world's most trusted authorities on unconventional medical treatments. Dr. Weil's sensible, interdisciplinary medical perspective strikes a strong chord in many people. His recent books are all *New York Times* bestsellers, and he has appeared on the cover of *Time Magazine* twice, in 1997 and again in 2005. *USA Today* said, "Clearly, Dr. Weil has hit a medical nerve," and the *New York Times Magazine* said, "Dr. Weil has arguably become America's best-known doctor."

Despite being in the limelight, Weil has always been outspoken about the benefits he gained from using psychedelics. I asked him how psychedelics have affected his perspective on medicine and what sort of therapeutic potential did he think they had. He replied:

I think they've been a very profound influence. I used them a lot when I was younger. I think that they made me very much aware, first of all, of the profound influence of consciousness on health. I have published and described one of the experiences that I had that was very dramatic, and this was seized upon by some networks that put it all out there. This was that I had become cured of a lifelong cat allergy. If a cat touched me I would get hives. If a cat licked me I would get hives and my eyes would swell. So I always avoided them. Then one day when I was twenty-eight I took LSD with some friends. It was a perfect day. I was in a wonderful state of mind, feeling totally relaxed and at one with everything, and a cat jumped into my lap. My immediate reaction was to be defensive, and then I instantly thought, *Well, here I'm in this state. Why don't I try to pet the cat?* So I petted the cat, and I had no allergic reaction. I spent a lot of time with it, and I've never had an allergic reaction to a cat since. So, to me, that's an example of a potential of those drugs, and if they were legally available I think that I would use them as teaching tools to show people that you can change chronic patterns of illness, because even if you aren't cured of an illness the psychedelic may show you that it's possible.

Another experience that I've written about with psychedelics is when I was learning yoga and had a lot of difficulty with some positions. The one I had the most trouble with was the Plow, where you lie on your back and try to touch your toes behind your head. I could get to about a foot off the floor and I had horrible pain in my neck. I had worked at this for weeks and made no progress. I was on the point of giving up, just thinking I was too old. I was twenty-eight then. I thought I was too old, that my body was too stiff. Again, an experience with a psychedelic, where I felt completely happy and elastic, showed me otherwise. I noticed that my body felt very free. So I tried that posture, and I thought I had around a foot left to go when my feet touched the floor and there was no pain. I kept raising and lowering them, and it was just delightful. The next day when I tried to do it I could get to a foot within the floor, and I had horrible pain in my neck—but there was a difference. I now knew that it was possible, and I think that's a model for how these drugs can work.

Psychedelics can show you possibilities. They don't give you information about how to maintain the experiences, and if you try to rely on the drug for the experience the drug stops working after a time. But in this case, just having seen that it was possible, I was motivated to keep working at it, and in a few weeks I was able to do it. I don't think I would have pursued that if I hadn't seen the possibility. So I think they're potentially tremendous teaching tools about mind-body interactions and states of consciousness.

SPIRITUALITY AND PSYCHEDELICS

In physician and author Deepak Chopra's book *How to Know God* he maps out the stages of spiritual evolution as he has come to understand them. In reading the book I was surprised that he didn't give any credibility to the psychedelic experience as being a genuine source of religious or spiritual insight. He mentioned it briefly and then seemed to swiftly dismiss it. I was surprised that he didn't give any credence to the work of people like Aldous Huxley, Alan Watts, Huston Smith, Ram Dass, Roland Griffiths, and many other important religious scholars and researchers who believe that psychedelic drugs like LSD, mescaline, and psilocybin can sometimes trigger powerful and authentic religious experiences. So I asked Chopra about this. I asked him if he ever had a psychedelic experience himself, and why he so quickly dismissed in his book the idea that psychedelics can sometimes trigger true religious experiences. He replied:

First of all, I grew up in a tradition that is so grounded in the understanding of consciousness that psychedelic experiences are considered hardly important—although in India, in rituals, we do occasionally use things like bhang, which is a form of marijuana, and mushrooms as well. I personally have used everything, including LSD, but that was when I was a medical student, more out of curiosity than anything else. And I do believe that these experiences can sometimes open a window to the transcendent and to the nonlocal domain of existence. I had a wonderful experience when I used them—but I was seventeen, and that was a long time ago. I didn't feel the need to rely on drugs, and, as a physician, I've met many people who have suffered from psychosis and other kinds of problems as a result of relying on drugs or psychedelic chemicals to have an experience.

As far as the work of Aldous Huxley, Alan Watts, Huston Smith, and Ram Dass goes, I think that they're very important religious scholars, and I believe what they're saying is very authentic. And I do think that they had great insights to give them a glimpse of this deeper reality. It just happens that I came from a tradition where this was almost taken for granted.

Spiritual teacher Ram Dass, who, along with Timothy Leary and Ralph Metzner, led research experiments with psychedelics at Harvard in the early 1960s, has been very outspoken about the benefits he gained from his personal use of psychedelics. When I asked him how his experience with psychedelics affected his view of life he replied:

It had no effect on me whatsoever, and nobody should use it! The predicament about history is that you keep rewriting the history. I'm not sure, as I look back, whether what appeared to be critical events are really as critical as I thought they were, because a lot of people took psychedelics and didn't have the reaction I had. That had something to do with everything that went before that moment. In a way I just see it as another event, but I can say that taking psychedelics and meeting my guru were the two most profound experiences in my life. Psychedelics helped me to escape—albeit momentarily—from the prison of my mind. It overrode the habit patterns of thought, and I was able to taste innocence again. Looking at sensations freshly, without the conceptual overlay was very profound.

Joan Halifax, Ph.D.—medical anthropologist, Zen priest, hospice caregiver, civil rights activist, ecologist, and renowned author—has an unusual talent for integrating scientific and spiritual disciplines. Halifax has done extensive work with the dying for more than forty years. In 1994 she founded the Project on Being with Dying, which has trained hundreds of health care professionals in the contemplative care of dying people. In the 1970s Halifax and her ex-husband, Stanislav

Grof, collaborated on a landmark LSD research project with terminally ill cancer patients at the Spring Grove Hospital in Maryland. When I interviewed Halifax I asked her how the LSD research that she did with Grof affected her perspective on death and dying. She replied:

Stan and I worked with dying people at the Maryland Psychiatric Research Center. Prior to this I had been at the University of Miami School of Medicine, where I saw that the most marginalized people in that medical setting were individuals who were dying. The physicians would say that medicine and drugs are about saving lives. So when Stan and I got married and I moved up to the Baltimore area, I joined him in his project, working with dying people. It was a very extraordinary project. It was really a contemporary rite of passage. I had studied rites of passage as an anthropologist, and to engage in such a powerful one was very interesting. So he and I worked with a number of people who were dying of cancer. Subjects were referred to the project by social workers and physicians. There was one patient, a doctor who had referred himself to the group. He was dying of pancreatic cancer, and through that work I had the opportunity to have a real experience in seeing that the human spirit, the human psyche, is profoundly underestimated.

LSD is referred to as an nonspecific amplifier of the psyche, and I felt very privileged to sit for many hours with a person dying of cancer and share his or her psyche in the most intimate way—aspects of which were, in general, not normally accessible in a nonaltered state of consciousness. It inspired me to continue the work. I began this work in 1970, feeling very concerned about dying people. Prior to that I'd been inspired by my grandmother who was taking care of dying people, and then herself had a very difficult death. I made a vow that I would try to make a difference. Then I saw that the work with LSD was so effective in facilitating a deep psychological process for people who were dying that it actually enhanced their quality of their life and their relationships. It enhanced their experience of dying and of death.

Medical marijuana and hospice activist Valerie Corral also spoke with me about how her experience with psychedelics influenced her perspective on life.

> It's been a profound tool for me, and generally people can say that—or not. I owe a lot to psychedelics. I think it opened my life and changed the possibilities for me. Although I had that altered experience that I described earlier, I might have gotten caught thinking that that was the only way—that there was a certain path, and then gotten caught in the path. Psychedelics helped me to see the vastness, the nondimensional, the altered-dimensional, and that it wasn't one way. It wasn't anyway single that I could see it. For me, it has been a tumbling of awareness, a tumbling out and through it. And again, probably the greatest and most significant possibility was really through allowance. It takes us out of the realm of being in control—so it's fabulous for all of us control freaks.

I was fortunate enough to be able to attend Swiss chemist (and LSD inventor) Albert Hofmann's one hundredth birthday celebration in Basel, Switzerland, in 2006. While I was there I asked him how his own use of LSD affected his philosophy of life. He responded simply by saying: "LSD showed me the inseparable interaction between the material and the spiritual world."

THE RELATIONSHIP BETWEEN CREATIVITY AND PSYCHEDELICS

I suspect that every creative person who has ever taken a psychedelic drug or plant yearns to express the experience, and one of the primary reasons why psychedelics influence culture so much is because they are known to enhance creativity. As we discussed in the introduction with cannabis and creativity, research studies by Willis Harman, James Fadiman, Oscar Janiger, and others have confirmed that something substantial underlies the claims made by many talented people that psychedelics can enhance their creative performance.

Psychiatrists Louis Berlin and Oscar Janiger demonstrated in studies of accomplished artists how mescaline and LSD could improve the creativity scores on the artists' paintings, and studies conducted by psychologist James Fadiman show how mescaline could enhance problem-solving skills among professionals from a variety of fields. In the first appendix to this book you'll find an essay that I wrote about the future of psychedelic drug research, where I review these studies and explore the creative potential of these agents in depth.

When I interviewed Janiger about creativity and psychedelics, he said:

> I studied the conditions under which people have these [creative] releases, breakthroughs, or have access to other ways and forms of perceiving the world around them and changing their reality. When I studied the works of people who profess to go to creative artists and ask them how they did it and what it was about, I realized that what we had by way of understanding creativity was a tremendous collection of highly idiosyncratic and subjective responses. There was no real way of dealing with the creative process as a state you could refer to across the board or how one could encourage it. That's how I got the idea for a study in which we could deliberately change consciousness in an artist using LSD, given the same reference object to paint before and during the experience. Then I would try to make an inference from the difference between the artwork outside of the drug experience and while they were having it.

The creativity studies that have been done with psychedelics provide compelling evidence that not only can LSD and other psychedelics significantly enhance the imagination, inspire novel thought, and strengthen problem-solving abilities, but they can also actually improve creativity and artistic performance. Because creativity lies at the heart of solving every problem that we face as a species, new studies in this area are desperately needed.

Personal growth, psychological transformation, ecological awareness, creativity, spirituality, psychic phenomena, and nonhuman-entity contact are just some of the critical areas that psychedelics are eager to teach us about. If we listen and learn from these powerful teachers with an open heart, an open mind, and with our eyes focused on the horizon—where the imagination meets the material world—we will forever find our new beginnings.

APPENDIX 1

Transcending the Medical Frontiers

Exploring the Future of Psychedelic Drug Research

When I was in graduate school studying behavioral neuroscience I wanted nothing more than to be able to conduct psychedelic drug research. However, in the mid-1980s this was impossible to do at any academic institution. There wasn't a single government on the entire planet that legally allowed clinical research with psychedelic drugs. But this worldwide research ban started to recede in the early 1990s, and we're currently witnessing a renaissance of medical research on psychedelic drugs.

Working with the Multidisciplinary Association for Psychedelic Studies (MAPS) for the past four years as their guest editor has been an extremely exciting and tremendously fruitful endeavor for me. It's a great joy to see how MDMA can help people suffering from post-traumatic stress disorder (PTSD), how LSD can help advanced-stage cancer patients come to peace with the dying process, and how ibogaine can help opiate addicts overcome their addiction. There appears to be enormous potential for the development of psychedelic drugs into effective treatments for a whole range of difficult-to-treat psychiatric disorders.

However, as thrilled as I am by all the new clinical studies exploring the medical potential of psychedelic drugs, I still long for the day when our best minds and resources can be applied to the study of these extraordinary substances with an eye that looks beyond their medical applications and toward their ability to enhance human potential and explore new realities.

This appendix explores these possibilities. But first let's take a look at how we got to be where we are.

A BRIEF HISTORY OF TIME-DILATION STUDIES

Psychedelic drug research began in 1897, when the German chemist Arthur Heffter first isolated mescaline, the primary psychoactive compound in the peyote cactus. In 1943 Swiss chemist Albert Hofmann discovered the hallucinogenic effects of LSD (lysergic acid diethylamide) at Sandoz Pharmaceuticals in Basel while studying ergot, a fungus that grows on rye. Then, fifteen years later in 1958, he was the first to isolate psilocybin and psilocin—the psychoactive components of the Mexican "magic mushroom," *Psilocybe mexicana.*

Before 1972 nearly seven hundred studies with LSD and other psychedelic drugs were conducted. This research suggested that LSD has remarkable medical potential. LSD-assisted psychotherapy was shown to safely reduce the anxiety of terminal cancer patients, the drinking of alcoholics, and the symptoms of many difficult-to-treat psychiatric illnesses.

Between 1972 and 1990 there were no human studies with psychedelic drugs. Their disappearance was the result of a political backlash that followed the promotion of these drugs by the 1960s counterculture. This reaction not only made these substances illegal for personal use but also made it extremely difficult for researchers to get government approval to study them.

THE NEW WAVE OF PSYCHEDELIC DRUG RESEARCH

The political climate began to change in 1990 with the approval of Rick Strassman's DMT study at the University of New Mexico. According to public-policy expert and MAPS president Rick Doblin this change occurred because "open-minded regulators at the FDA decided to put science before politics when it came to psychedelic and medical marijuana research. FDA openness to research is really the key factor. Also, senior researchers who were influenced by psychedelics in the sixties now are speaking up before they retire and have earned credibility."

The past eighteen years have seen a bold resurgence of psychedelic drug research as scientists all over the world have come to recognize the long-underappreciated potential of these drugs. In the past few years a growing number of studies using human volunteers have begun to explore the possible therapeutic benefits of drugs such as LSD, psilocybin, DMT, MDMA, ibogaine, and ketamine.

Current studies are focusing on psychedelic treatments for cluster headaches, PTSD, depression, obsessive-compulsive disorder (OCD), severe anxiety in terminal cancer patients, alcoholism, and opiate addiction. The results so far look quite promising, and more studies are being planned by MAPS and other private psychedelic research organizations, with the eventual goal of turning MDMA, LSD, psilocybin, and other psychedelics into legally available prescription drugs.

As excited as I am that psychedelic drugs are finally being studied for their medical and healing potential, I'm eagerly anticipating the day when psychedelic drug research can really take off and move beyond its therapeutic applications in medicine. I look forward to the day when researchers can explore the potential of psychedelics as advanced learning tools, relationship builders, creativity enhancers, pleasure magnifiers, vehicles for self-improvement, reliable catalysts for spiritual or mystical experiences, a stimulus for telepathy and other psychic abilities, windows into other dimensions, and for their ability to possibly shed light on the reality of parallel universes and nonhuman-entity contact.

Let's take a look at some of these exciting possibilities.

THE SCIENCE OF PLEASURE

Almost all of the medical research with psychedelic drugs to date has been focused on curing diseases and treating illnesses. Despite countless anecdotal reports, and a few encouraging pilot studies, little attention has been paid to the reported ability of these remarkable substances to increase human potential, and even less attention has been paid to their reputed ability to significantly enhance all aspects of human pleasure.

However, one can envision a time in the not-too-distant future when we will have cured our most challenging pathological conditions and have more time and resources on our hands to explore post-survival activities. It's likely that we'll then focus our research efforts on discovering new ways to improve our physical and mental performance. A science devoted purely to enhancing pleasure might come next, and psychedelics could play a major role in this new field.

According to surveys done by the U.S. National Institute of Drug Abuse, the number one reason why people use LSD is because "it's fun." Tim Leary helped to popularize the use of LSD with the help of the word "ecstasy," and sex expert Annie Sprinkle has been outspoken about the ecstatic possibilities available from combining sex and psychedelics.

Many hundreds of psychedelic trip reports have described long periods of deeply appreciating extraordinary beauty and savoring ecstatic bliss, experiences that were many orders of magnitude more intense than the subjects previously thought possible.

With all the current research emphasis on the medical applications and therapeutic potential of psychedelics, in research circles the unspoken and yet obvious truth about these extraordinary substances is that, when done properly, they're generally safe and healthy ways to have an enormous amount of fun. There's good reason why they're so popular recreationally, despite being illegal.

When psychedelic research begins to integrate with applied neuroscience and advanced nanotechnology in the future, we can begin to establish a serious science of pleasure and fun. Most likely this would begin with a study of sensory enhancement and time dilation (slowing down the perception of time), which are two of the primary effects that psychedelic drugs reliably produce.

Perhaps one day our brightest researchers and best resources will be devoted to finding new ways to enhance sexual, auditory, visual, olfactory, gustatory, and tactile sensations, and create undreamed of new pleasures and truly unearthly delights.

Scientific studies could explore new and better ways to improve sexual performance and further enhance sensory sensitivity, elongate and intensify our orgasms, enlarge the spectrum of our perceptions, and deepen every dimension of our experience.

Massage therapy, Tantra, music, culinary crafting, and other pleasure-producing techniques and activities could be systematically explored with psychedelics, and universities could have applied research centers devoted to the study of ecstasy, tickling, and laughter.

The neurochemistry of aesthetic appreciation, happiness, humor, euphoria, and bliss could be carefully explored with an eye toward improvement. Serious research and development could be used to create new drugs and integrate neurochemically heightened states with enhanced environments, such as nanotechnologically advanced amusement parks and super-realistic virtual realities.

In this area of research it seems that psychedelic drugs may prove to be extremely useful, and countless new psychedelic drugs are just waiting to be discovered.

According to a 2012 paper by chemists Jean-Louis Reymond and Mahendra Awale, "Exploring Chemical Space for Drug Discovery Using the Chemical Universe Database" in the American Chemical Society's journal *Chemical Neuroscience*, scientists have synthesized barely one-tenth of 1 percent of the potential drugs that could be made. This paper esti-mates that the actual number of "small molecule" medicines could be around one novemdecillion—one million billion billion billion billion billion billion—which is more than some estimates of the number of stars in the universe.

Maverick physicist Nick Herbert has suggested diverting a portion of the U.S. military budget to fund the creation of a series of "pleasure domes." Herbert's "Pleasure Dome" project seeks to explore the possi-bilities of amplifying pleasure, and although this project is little more than an idea at this point, it may be the first step toward turning the enhancement of pleasure into a true science.

In addition to enhancing pleasure, psychedelics also stimulate the imagination in extraordinary ways.

CREATIVITY AND PROBLEM SOLVING

A number of early studies suggest that psychedelic drugs may stimulate creativity and improve problem-solving abilities. In 1955 Louis Berlin investigated the effects of mescaline and LSD on the painting abili-ties of four nationally recognized graphic artists. Although the study showed that there was some impairment of technical ability among the artists, a panel of independent art critics judged the experimental paint-ings as having greater aesthetic value than the artists' usual work.

In 1959 Los Angeles psychiatrist Oscar Janiger asked sixty promi-nent artists to paint a Native American doll before taking LSD and then again while under its influence. These 120 paintings were then evaluated by a panel of independent art critics and historians. As with Berlin's study, there was a general agreement by the judges that the craftsmanship of the LSD paintings suffered; however, many received higher marks for imagination than the pre-LSD paintings.

In 1965 James Fadiman and Willis Harman at San Francisco State University administered mescaline to professional workers in various fields to explore its creative problem-solving abilities. The subjects were instructed to bring a professional problem requiring a creative solution to their sessions. After some psychological preparation, subjects worked individually on their problem throughout their mescaline session. The creative output of each subject was evaluated by psychological tests, subjective reports, and the eventual industrial or commercial validation and acceptance of the finished product or final solution. Virtually all subjects produced solutions judged highly creative and satisfactory by these standards. These studies are summarized and explored in detail in James Fadiman's book *The Psychedelic Explorer's Guide.*

In addition to the scientific studies that have been conducted there are also a number of compelling anecdotal examples that suggest a link between creativity and psychedelic drugs. For example, architect Kyosho Izumi's LSD-inspired design of the ideal psychiatric hospital won him a commendation for outstanding achievement from the American Psychiatric Association, and the late Apple cofounder Steve Jobs attributed some of the insights that led to the development of the personal computer to his use of LSD. Additionally, a number of renowned scientists have personally attributed their breakthrough scientific insights to their use of psychedelic drugs—including Nobel Prize winners Francis Crick and Kary Mullis.

There hasn't been a formal creativity study with psychedelics since 1965, although there are countless anecdotal reports of artists, writers, musicians, filmmakers, and other people who attribute a portion of their creativity and inspiration to their use of psychedelics. This is an area that is more than ripe for study. Anecdotal reports suggest that very low doses of LSD—threshold-level doses, around 20 micrograms—are especially effective as creativity enhancers. For example, Francis Crick was reported to have used low doses of LSD when he discovered the double-helix structure of the DNA molecule.

I'd love to see a whole series of new studies exploring how cannabis, LSD, psilocybin, and mescaline can enhance the imagination, improve problem-solving abilities, and stimulate creativity. At the time of this writing the Beckley Foundation in England is supporting a study into the effects of cannabis on creativity, which I discussed in the introduction, and is getting positive results. As more and more of our world becomes automated with advanced robotics, I suspect that creativity will eventually become the most valuable commodity of all. Much of the creativity in Hollywood and the Silicon Valley is already fueled by psychedelics, and research into how these extraordinary tools could enhance creativity even more effectively may become a booming enterprise in the not-too-distant future.

However, creativity isn't the only valuable psychological ability that psychedelics appear to enhance.

ESP AND PSYCHIC PHENOMENA

Few people are aware that there have been numerous, carefully controlled scientific experiments with telepathy, psychokinesis, remote viewing, and other types of psychic phenomena, which have consistently produced compelling, statistically significant results that conventional science is at a loss to explain. Even most scientists are currently unaware of the vast abundance of compelling scientific evidence for psychic phenomena, which has resulted from more than a century of parapsychological research.

Hundreds of carefully controlled studies—in which psi researchers continuously redesigned experiments to address the comments from their critics—have produced results that demonstrate small but statistically significant effects for psi phenomena, such as telepathy, precognition, and psychokinesis.

According to Dean Radin a meta-analysis of this research demonstrates that the positive results from these studies are significant with odds in the order of many billions to one. Princeton University, the SRI International, Duke University, the Institute of Noetic Sciences, the U.S. and Russian governments, and many other respectable institutions have spent years researching these mysterious phenomena, and conventional science is at a loss to explain the results. This research is summarized in Radin's remarkable book *The Conscious Universe*.

Just as fascinating as the research into psychic phenomena is the controversy that surrounds it. In my own experience researching the possibility of telepathy in animals and other unexplained phenomena with British biologist Rupert Sheldrake, I discovered that many people are eager to share personal anecdotes about psychic events in their life—such as remarkable coincidences, uncanny premonitions, precognitive dreams, and seemingly telepathic communications. In these cases the scientific studies simply confirm life experiences. Yet many scientists with whom I've spoken haven't reviewed the evidence and remain doubtful that there is any reality to psychic phenomenon. However, surveys conducted by Sheldrake and me reveal that around 78 percent of the population has had unexplainable psychic experiences, and the scientific evidence supports the validity of these experiences.

It's also interesting to note that many people have reported experiencing meaningful psychic experiences with psychedelics—not to mention a wide range of paranormal events and synchronicities that seem extremely difficult to explain by means of conventional reasoning.

Psychologist Charles Tart, Ph.D., conducted a questionnaire study of 150 experienced marijuana users and found that 76 percent believed in extrasensory perception (ESP), with frequent reports of experiences while they were high. Psychiatrist Stanislav Grof, M.D., and psychologist Stanley Krippner, Ph.D., have collected numerous anecdotes about psychic phenomena that were reported by people under the influence of psychedelics, and several small scientific studies have looked at how LSD, psilocybin, and mescaline might affect telepathy and remote viewing.

For example, according to psychologist Jean Millay, Ph.D., in 1997 students at the University of Amsterdam in the Netherlands did research to establish whether the use of psilocybin could influence remote viewing. This was a small experiment, with only twelve test subjects, but the results of the study indicated that subjects who were under the influence of psilocybin achieved a success rate of 58.3 percent, which was statistically significant.

A new edition of the 1964 book *ESP Experiments with LSD-25 and*

Psilocybin: A Methodological Approach, by Roberto Cavanna and Emilio Servadio, was republished in 2010 with a new preface by Charles Tart. In the introduction Tart states that "this study remains as important today as when it was first published, and will hopefully guide a new generation of researchers to finding the knowledge we need!"

A great review article by Krippner and psychologist David Luke, Ph.D., that summarizes all of the psychedelic research into psychic phenomena can be found in the spring 2011 *MAPS Bulletin* about psychedelics and the mind/body connection, which I edited. This article can be found at www.maps.org/news-letters/v21n1, starting on page 59. Also see Stanislav Grof's extraordinary book *When the Impossible Happens: Adventures in Non-Ordinary Realities* for a wonderful collection of psychedelic and paranormal anecdotes.

When I conducted the California-based research for two of Sheldrake's books about unexplained phenomena in science, *Dogs That Know When Their Owners Are Coming Home* and *The Sense of Being Stared At,* one of the experiments that I ran involved testing blindfolded subjects to see if they could sense being stared at from behind. One of the subjects I worked with reported an unusually high number of correct trials while under the influence of MDMA. I'd love to run a whole study to see if MDMA-sensitized subjects are more aware of when they're being stared at.

It is especially common for people to report experiences with telepathy, clairvoyance, precognition, remote viewing, and psychokinesis while using ayahuasca, the potent hallucinogenic jungle juice from the Amazon. In fact, when the chemical structure of an important psychoactive component of ayahuasca was first discovered, now called "harmaline," one of the original suggestions for its name was "telepathine," due to the psychedelic brew's common association with telepathy.

There have been several studies with ayahuasca that demonstrate health benefits, but this is an area that is just crying out to be explored carefully and in depth. Future studies could examine ayahuasca's potential and accuracy as a catalyst for psychic phenomena, and all of the traditional studies that have been done with psychic phenomena that generated positive results could be redone with subjects dosed with different psychedelics to see if test scores can be improved.

Increasing our psychic abilities may open the human mind to new, unimagined possibilities—and if you think that harnessing telepathic and clairvoyant abilities is pretty wild, then hold on to your hats for what's likely to come next.

HIGHER DIMENSIONS AND
NONHUMAN-ENTITY CONTACT

A primary ingredient in ayahuasca is DMT, and it appears that this remarkable substance has the extraordinary power to open an interdimensional portal into another universe. Some of the most fascinating psychedelic research has been done with this incredible compound.

As we discussed in chapter 4, DMT is a mystery, one of the strangest puzzles in all of nature. Psychiatric researcher Rick Strassman, Ph.D., who conducted a five-year study with DMT at the University of New Mexico, has suggested that naturally elevated DMT levels in the brain may be responsible for such unexplained mental phenomena as spontaneous mystical experiences, near-death experiences, nonhuman-entity contact, and schizophrenia. Strassman and others have even gone so far as to speculate about the possibility that elevated DMT levels in the brain might be responsible for ushering the soul into the body before birth and out of the body after death.

But perhaps what's most interesting about DMT is that, with great consistency, it appears to allow human beings to communicate with other intelligent life-forms. When I interviewed Strassman, I asked him if he thought that there was an objective reality to the worlds visited by people when they're under the influence of DMT, and if he thought that the entities that so many people have encountered on DMT actually have an independent existence. Rick replied, "I myself think so. My colleagues think I've gone woolly-brained over this, but I think it's as good a working hypothesis as any other."

A 2006 scientific paper by computer scientist Marko A. Rodriguez called "A Methodology for Studying Various Interpretations of the N,N-dimethyltryptamine-Induced Alternate Reality" explores how to possibly determine if the entities experienced by people on DMT are indeed independently existing, intelligent beings or just projections of our hallucinating brains. Rodriguez suggests a test that involves asking the entities to perform a complex mathematical task involving prime numbers to verify their independent existence. While it seems like a long shot that this method could lead to fruitful results, I think that any serious speculation about establishing communication channels with these mysterious beings is constructive.

Strassman's work could represent the very beginning of a scientific field that systematically explores the possibility of communicating with higher-dimensional entities, and this might prove to be a more fruitful endeavor for establishing extraterrestrial contact than the SETI project. What they can teach us we can only imagine.

My own experiences with DMT led me to suspect that Strassman's studies would have yielded far more useful results had the subjects been dosed with harmaline prior to receiving their DMT injections. Harmaline is an MAO-inhibiting enzyme that is found in a number of plants. It's found in the famous South American vine known as *Banisteriopsis caapi,* which composes half the mixture in the sacred hallucinogenic jungle juice ayahuasca, which has been used for healing purposes by indigenous peoples in the Amazon basin for thousands of years. Harmaline is widely known as the chemical that allows the DMT in other plants, like *Psychotria viridis,* to become orally active.

Orally consumed DMT is destroyed in the stomach by an enzyme called monoamine oxidase (MAO), which harmaline inhibits. However, it does much more than just make the DMT orally active. I've discovered that drinking a tea made from Syrian rue seeds, which also contain harmaline, two hours prior to smoking DMT dramatically alters the experience. Harmaline has interesting psychoactive properties of its own that are somewhat psychedelic, and it slows down the speed of the DMT experience considerably, rendering it more comprehensible and less frightening. For thousands of years indigenous peoples in the Amazon jungles combined harmaline and DMT, and this long history has cultivated a powerful synergism between how the two molecules react in our body.

In future studies harmaline could be used in conjunction with DMT to more accurately simulate the ayahuasca experience that strikes such a powerful primordial chord in our species. This would allow the experience to become not only much easier to understand but also to last for a greater duration of time, which would allow for more ability to examine the phenomenon of nonhuman-entity communication.

Some astute readers may have noticed that this appendix has loosely followed a Christian theological progression, from the ego death and bodily resurrection of the medical studies with psychedelics to the paradisical pleasures of Heaven, where we discovered our godlike powers and met with the angels. Ultimately, it appears, this research will lead us to the source of divinity itself.

THE STUDY OF DIVINE INTELLIGENCE

Perhaps the most vital function of psychedelics is their ability to reliably produce spiritual or mystical experiences. These transpersonal experiences of inseparability often result in an increased sense of ecological awareness, a greater sense of interconnection, a transcendence of the fear of death, a sense of the sacred or divine, and an identification with something much larger than one's body or personal life.

Many people suspect that this experience lies at the heart of the healing potential of psychedelics, and that making this experience available to people is essential for the survival of our species. I agree that we need a compassionate vision of our interconnection with the biosphere to guide our technological evolution, or we appear doomed to destroy ourselves.

In his book *The Physics of Immortality,* physicist Frank Tipler introduces the idea that if a conscious designing intelligence is genuinely a part of this universe, then ultimately religion—or the study of this designer intelligence—will become a branch of physics. Psychedelic drug research may offer one pathway toward establishing this science of the future.

Recent studies by Roland Griffiths and colleagues at Johns Hopkins University have confirmed that psilocybin can indeed cause religious experiences—which are indistinguishable from religious experiences reported by mystics throughout the ages—and that substantial health benefits can result from these experiences.

These new studies echo the findings of an earlier study done in 1962 by Walter Pahnke of the Harvard Divinity School, and it's certainly not news to anyone who has had a full-blown psychedelic experience. R.U. Sirius responded to this seemingly redundant research by saying, "Wow! Scientists Discover Ass, Not Elbow!" Nonetheless, this may represent the beginning of a whole new field of academic inquiry, which explores those realms that have been previously declared off-limits to science.

It appears that the integration of science and spirituality lies on the horizon of our adventure as a species and that our future evolution depends on this. Without a transpersonal perspective of interconnection to guide our evolutionary direction, we seem to be firmly set on a path toward inevitable self-destruction. I think that psychedelics can help us get back on track and help us heal the damage that we've done to ourselves and to the Earth. This is why I believe so strongly in psychedelic drug research.

There isn't much time left before our biosphere starts to unravel, and we may have only a small window of opportunity to save our fragile world. I think that MAPS and sister organizations like the Beckley Foundation and the Heffter Research Institute are industrialized society's best hope for transforming the planet's ancient shamanic plants into the respectable scientific medicines of tomorrow and, in so doing, bring psychedelic therapy to all who need it. This may not only help to heal a number of difficult-to-treat medical disorders and increase ecological harmony on the planet, but it may also open up a doorway to untold and unimagined new worlds of possibility.

INTERVIEWS WITH DAVID JAY BROWN

Seeing as I've spent so much of my life conducting interviews, I think that it's only fair to have the tables turned on me. What follows are two interviews that some talented journalists conducted with me. —DJB

The Man Behind
Mavericks of the Mind

An Interview with David Jay Brown

By Ian Koslow from Time-Peace

This interview was conducted by Ian Koslow on October 14, 2010. It appears on the Time-Peace Facebook page.

Your journey begins the moment you realize you're on it. For us that journey started long before Time-Peace, and along the way came a handful of books that helped pave the way. One of those books was *Mavericks of the Mind,* a collection of interviews from some of the most original thinkers and leading-edge philosophers in the world.

   Now, in anticipation of the release of the new edition of *Mavericks of the Mind,* we had the opportunity to interview the man who made it all possible. For those of you who have read his books, you know how cool he is. And for those of you who haven't, it's an honor for us to introduce you to David Jay Brown. —Ian Koslow

TP: What did you hope to achieve when you first created *Mavericks of the Mind*? Looking back, what would you say you have achieved?

DJB: When Rebecca and I first began doing interviews together back in 1989, we wanted to ask leading-edge thinkers important questions that few people were asking them in interviews. We were particularly interested in philosophical questions about the nature of reality and consciousness and about the interface between science, creativity, and spirituality. Our fascination with these topics had emerged from our late-night, cannabis-fueled discussions and our occasional psychedelic journeys together.

We were actually pretty surprised that nobody had really interviewed all these brilliant thinkers about these philosophical topics before. We were interested in questions like: How did consciousness arise? What happens to consciousness after death? Will the human species survive, and, if so, how will humans evolve in the future? What is the nature of God? What inspires creativity? How is technology affecting human evolution and human consciousness? How have psychedelics affected your work and your perspective on life?

We asked these questions to pretty much everyone we interviewed and combined them with personal questions about their work and questions about one another's work. One of the key things that Rebecca and I initially set out to do with these interviews was to foster interaction and exchange between our interviewees. We wanted to create a more inclusive perspective, one that combined their viewpoints into a larger whole. This was the single most important goal of *Mavericks of the Mind,* and we tried to synergize what we believed were the most important messages emerging on the planet.

I think that we achieved these lofty goals with the book rather well, and looking back I can see how the book served a valuable function by concisely summarizing some unusually valuable ideas and introducing them to a new audience. I've received many letters from people over the years who told me that the book was inspirational to them at key points in their lives, that learning about certain ideas in the book helped to change their perspective, and that the book played an important role in inspiring a number of people to explore the ideas presented in the book further.

TP: You've interviewed some the greatest thinkers of our lifetime. So we're curious: if you could interview anyone from any time period in the history of the world, who would it be?

DJB: Great question! Actually, I enjoy consulting with historical figures all the time while I'm meditating in altered states of consciousness, as an exercise of the imagination. But, really, there are just too many incredible historical figures I'd like to interview, and to pick a single one would just be too difficult. So I'll mention a few people who come to mind. Some of the people I wish I had been able to interview include John Lennon, Aldous Huxley, Ken Kesey, Alan Watts, Cary Grant, William Burroughs, Socrates, Robert Crumb, and Herman Hesse.

TP: Out of all the interviews you've done, is there one that stands out among the rest? How about the best answer you've ever received?

DJB: Oh, that's a really tough question to answer. There are a couple of interviews that really stand out for me and were especially magical and fun to conduct. I'd say that the interviews with John Lilly, Jerry Garcia, Matthew Fox, and George Carlin were among my favorites. I think that my all-time favorite response came from a question to Terence McKenna. I asked Terence what he thought the ultimate goal of human evolution was, and he replied, "Oh, a good party."

TP: One of our favorites is definitely John C. Lilly. One question you always ask is about death and whether it is believed consciousness continues to exist beyond the body. Do you think Lilly looked at death as the ultimate sensory deprivation?

DJB: That's an interesting question, and I'm not really sure how John would respond to that. John was a real trickster, and I would take everything that he said with a grain of salt, because it was sometimes difficult to tell when he was being serious and when he was being playful. John did sometimes talk about certain parallels between his ketamine trips in the isolation tank and what he thought happened to consciousness after death. However, he also said that he refused to equate his experiences with death, and he seemed to be content with the mystery. However, I remember Tim Leary once saying something about death that I think relates to your question. He said that death isn't really all that hard to imagine when you think about how alive you are right now in faraway places, and, at the time, he seemed to be implying that death might just be a loss of sensory data.

TP: Another topic you love to ask about is lucid dreaming. Do you see any parallels between this "evolution of consciousness" taking place and a sort of collective waking up from within the dream world?

DJB: Yes, indeed. I think that's a really good metaphor for what's going on. I suspect that all matter and energy in the universe is ultimately composed of consciousness and that the final goal of evolution is for the external world of material reality to fully mirror the internal world of the collective imagination. I suspect that dreams and realities are, ultimately, just different levels, vibrational states, or dimensions of the same world and that both are just as real or unreal as the other. It seems to me as though most people are sleepwalking through their lives and that our culture puts us into a kind of trance. Becoming more conscious and understanding that we're continuously creating reality and shaping it with our own minds is the first step, I think, toward waking up from the trancelike slumber that we're in and taking a more formative role in the creation of reality.

TP: It must be a bit funny being on the other side of the interview process. What question would you ask yourself that we would never think of?

DJB: Well, I'm not sure that I can think of something to ask myself that you would never think of, but I can try. I guess that I would ask myself the following question, as this is something that's really been on my mind a lot lately: Do I think that the hyperdimensional, transcorporeal beings that one encounters on a powerful shamanic journey with ayahuasca or DMT have a freestanding, independent existence, or are they merely parts of my own psyche? This is something that I've thought about quite a bit, in various states of consciousness, and have discussed in detail with various experts—like DMT researcher Rick Strassman, anthropologist Jeremy Narby, and the late ethnobotanist Terence McKenna—and I still haven't really got a clue as to what is going on. I think the answer may lie in transcending the black-and-white nature of the question and understanding that there may be other possibilities besides dividing the whole universe into "self" and "other."

TP: Who is the ultimate Maverick of the Mind, or what makes someone a maverick of the mind?

DJB: A maverick is basically an independent thinker, someone who thinks for him- or herself, and all my illustrious interviewees are experts in various fields who have all given some thought to the evolution of consciousness and the exploration of the mind. There are quintessential mavericks of the mind—such as Timothy Leary, Terence McKenna, Robert Anton Wilson, and John Lilly—although I think that any kind of ultimate maverick of the mind would have to be some kind of transpersonal being, a composite or a community of people. I guess the ultimate maverick of the mind is the composite being that's created by integrating the interdisciplinary views of all our different interviewees.

TP: What an amazing opportunity it is to have learned from some of the most brilliant beings on the planet. Although they all have different ideas and perspectives, do you find any one overarching theme that unites all of their philosophies together?

DJB: Not so much one overarching theme, I don't think, but several cross-pollinating themes—such as interconnection; the integration of science and spirituality; transcending culture; being comfortable with mystery; and the necessity for compassionate, creative, and conscious thinking. We really tried to create a synergistic perspective with *Mavericks of the Mind* by linking together the ideas and concepts of those people we interviewed. This interconnecting thread that runs through the interviews demonstrates that the visions expressed—which stem from divergent points of view—are also complementary with one another, and this provides me with a tremendous sense of inspiration and hope.

TP: True or false? a) Time is an illusion.

DJB: In general, for all of the true-or-false questions I'd have to answer: sometimes true, sometimes false, sometimes true and false, and sometimes neither true or false. It all depends on one's context and state of consciousness.

That said, time and space are part of a continuum that can be transcended. Once transcended time and space then appear to be an illusion, in the sense that their perception depends on arbitrary distinctions and comparative movements.

TP: b) Your perception creates your reality.

DJB: You know, I can never seem to figure out if my perceptions create reality or vice versa. I think it's some kind of a back-and-forth process that continually feeds back on itself.

TP: c) Everything is interconnected.

DJB: I think that using the word *is* can be dangerous. Everything certainly appears to be fluidly interconnected, from both a scientific and a psychedelic perspective, although in normal, left-brain-dominated, waking consciousness boundaries appear, distinctions are drawn, and things appear to be quite separate. I'm not really sure what *is,* just how some things appear.

TP: d) The universe is in alignment.

DJB: Alignment with the multiverse? Wouldn't this require something outside of the universe for it to be in alignment with? I don't think that it can really ever possibly get out of alignment because it's always a perfect balance of positive and negative forces.

TP: If you had one last chance to tell everyone in the world one last thing, what would it be?

DJB: Nothing is more important than love. Please be kind to one another and don't take life so damn seriously.

Ian Koslow is a cofounder of Time-Peace, an innovative watch company aimed toward helping people to stop worrying and start Being.

APPENDIX 3

Altered Statesman

An Interview with David Jay Brown

By Damon Orion from *Good Times*

This interview with me by Damon Orion appeared as the cover story in the April 15, 2011, issue of Santa Cruz's entertainment weekly *Good Times*. That same year I was voted Best Writer in Santa Cruz in the annual *Good Times* Best of Santa Cruz poll.

Local psychedelic visionary David Jay Brown has peered deeply into the nature of human awareness, bonded with the greatest thinkers of our time and explored the outer limits of philosophy, science, spirituality and parapsychology. In this mind-expanding interview with *GT,* he shares tales from his journeys to the fringes of consciousness.

Consciousness: What is it? Are your thoughts and emotions nothing more than neural static? Will your physical death extinguish your awareness? Is your individual consciousness just one of innumerable facets of a universal consciousness?

In search of answers to questions like these, local writer/neuroscience researcher David Jay Brown has mind-melded with many of the world's most prominent philosophers, visionaries, culture-shapers and snorkelers of the psyche, including Timothy Leary, Terence McKenna, Robert Anton Wilson, Noam Chomsky, Ram Dass, Albert Hofmann, Jack Kevorkian, George Carlin, Sasha Shulgin, Deepak Chopra, Alex Grey,

Jerry Garcia, Stanislav Grof and John Lilly. He's chronicled these meetings in his bestselling interview compendiums *Conversations on the Edge of the Apocalypse, Mavericks of the Mind, Mavericks of Medicine* and *Voices from the Edge*. Dubbed "the most compelling interviewer on the planet" by author Clifford Pickover, Brown is currently working on an interview collection/psychedelic memoir called *Over the Edge of the Mind*.

Brown (mavericksofthemind.com; myspace.com/davidjaybrown; sexanddrugs.info) is also the author of the sci-fi books *Brainchild* and *Virus: The Alien Strain* and coauthor of the health book *Detox with Oral Chelation*. He frequently serves as guest editor of the tri-annual bulletin from the Multidisciplinary Association for Psychedelic Studies (MAPS), a local psychedelic research organization that recently published the second edition of *Mavericks of the Mind* (available at Bookshop Santa Cruz). He has written for periodicals such as *Mondo 2000, Scientific American Mind, Wired, High Times, The Sun, Magical Blend* and the *Journal of Psychical Research*. The diversity of his output is telling of his leave-no-stone-unturned approach to consciousness exploration: It's a good bet he's the only writer in history who's contributed to both the Buddhist wisdom publication *Tricycle* and the porn magazine *Hustler*.

Brown's studies of learning and memory at the University of Southern California in the early '80s earned him a B.A. in psychology. Between 1985 and 1986, he did research on electrical brain stimulation at New York University, obtaining a master's degree in psychobiology. His inquiries eventually led him into the realm of parapsychology: He's the man behind the California-based research for biologist Rupert Sheldrake's books *Dogs That Know When Their Owners Are Coming Home* and *The Sense of Being Stared At,* both of which presented scientific studies of unexplained phenomena. Brown's knowledge of such mysteries, as well as of technology, smart drugs, health, psychedelic research and sex-drug interaction, have landed him guest spots on shows like HBO's *Real Sex,* Fox's *A Current Affair,* PBS's *Nature,* ViaCom's *The Montel Williams Show* and the BBC and Discovery Channel's *Animal X.*

Journey with us, if you will, through the labyrinth of Mr. Brown's mind. . . .

DAMON: Tell me about the electrical brain stimulation research you've done.

DAVID: When I was at New York University, I did research for years where I surgically implanted electrical stimulating probes into the lateral hypothalamus of rats, which is a pleasure center. I would watch rats press a bar that delivered an electric current into their brain center over and over and over again until they fell asleep from exhaustion. Then they would wake up, and there was food sitting next to them, water sitting next to them, and a mate sitting next to them. They ignored all three and would continue to press that bar over and over again to get the reward stimulation over survival instincts. The other area of research I was involved in was at University of Southern California, and it was the exact opposite of the research I did at NYU, where I was surgically implanting electrodes into the brain centers of mammals and stimulating them: In this case I was inserting cold probes, which are devices that actually freeze or inhibit a certain part of the brain temporarily, so you can see how the animal operates with that one part of the brain missing, and how they operate when that part of the brain comes back. The anesthetic that we gave to the rabbits prior to surgery was a drug called ketamine. I took some of this ketamine home and experimented on myself with it. After injecting 50 milligrams of ketamine chloride into my right thigh muscle and turning the lights out, I suddenly "realized" that my professors and my fellow researchers and colleagues at USC were in reality extraterrestrials—that they were scientists who were there not to study rabbits; they were there to study me. I was the test subject, and they'd left this bottle of ketamine out for me to take. They were watching me right at this moment with a video camera. And suddenly I found myself in a cage with cold probes implanted in my brain and giant rabbits all around me. They were measuring me, and I was naked and helpless. Suddenly,

I snapped back into my body. I did not continue very much longer in that program after experiencing what I was experiencing from the rabbit's point of view. That's what ketamine taught me: what the rabbit was experiencing from what I was doing.

DAMON: You often ask your interviewees what they think happens to consciousness after death. If you had to put money on what happens after death, what would you bet on?

DAVID: I guess wherever you go after death, the money's not going to matter anymore! [Laughs.] You know, I think about that question every day, as an exercise of the imagination, and I change my mind about it all the time. I used to debate with my friend Nina Graboi—whom I interviewed for my book *Mavericks of the Mind,* and who passed away about 10 years ago—all the time about what happens to consciousness after death. It was one of our favorite topics of conversation. In general, I took the position that after you die, your individuality leaves, and your sense of awareness merges with the higher consciousness, the oneness, the source that everything came from originally. And her position was, "Well, there is that, but then there are all these levels in between where individuality remains besides the body, and you go through [multiple] incarnations with that. For years we went back and forth with this. Nina referred to her body as a spacesuit, and she always said she was going to get a new spacesuit when she died; she would go from one spacesuit to another. Well, after Nina died, I was writing in my journal, and the TV was on in the background. I was thinking about what was going on in Nina's mind when she was dying: "I'll bet she was thinking, 'Now I see: David Jay Brown was right! You do just merge with the one consciousness.'" As I'm sitting there in this kind of self-congratulatory way, I look at the television screen, and there on the TV screen were just two words: SPACE SUIT. There was this tingle up my spine; I stopped in my tracks; my jaw dropped open. It was the most profound sense of communication with somebody after they died that I'd ever experienced. That is the most compelling evidence I've experienced that consciousness not only continues [after death], but that some sense of individuality continues as well.

DAMON: What are your memories of your friend Timothy Leary?

DAVID: Well, my fondest and most important memories of Tim, I think, are [of] while he was dying. The last year [of his life], he announced to the media that he was thrilled and ecstatic that he was dying. And for the last year, while he was dying from prostate cancer, there was continuous celebration, continuous parties, continuously people coming around his house to tell him how important his work was to them. There was such a feeling of festivity and celebration and Tim deliberately trying to be playful and have fun with this process. This really made a very, very deep impression on me, because I ask so many questions about death—it's an important philosophical topic for me. And there have been so many people throughout history trying to die bravely or courageously or nobly, but before Tim, I don't think anybody ever tried to say, "Let's make dying fun!" [Laughs.] Tim really tried to party through the dying process, and I thought it was just a stroke of brilliance. I cried when he died; as much fun as it was, it was terribly sad the moment that he really left. But he just left us all with such a great message, I think.

DAMON: Tell me about your connection to Robert Anton Wilson.

DAVID: Bob was not only one of my closest friends, but he was the person who actually inspired me to become a writer. It was at the age of 16 that I read *Cosmic Trigger*, and that was how I encountered Timothy Leary, John Lilly and a number of the other people I went on to interview. I went to a lecture that Bob gave here in Santa Cruz back in the late '80s. At the end of the lecture, I went over to talk to him. I told him I was working on a book, and I asked him if he would possibly consider writing a blurb for the back cover. He kind of hemmed and hawed and looked not terribly enthusiastic, like I was the 15th person that day who asked him that, you know? [Laughs.] But he did tell me to have my publisher send him a copy of my book, and he would take a look at it. So you could only imagine my absolute delight when I discovered from my publisher that he ended up writing an 11-page introduction to my first book, *Brainchild*. It was through that that I became friends with him. He was a tremendous friend and mentor. When I had difficulty paying my rent early in my writing career, he actually sent me money to pay my rent! He was always there when I called him, giving me great advice. When an editor made some kind of change to one of my articles that I wasn't happy with, [he said,] "Editors don't like the way the soup tastes until they pee in it themselves." [Laughs.]

DAMON: What was your experience as a guest on *The Montel Williams Show*?

DAVID: I was on Montel Williams' show back in the early '90s, during his first season. There was all this anti-drug hysteria, and I was on the show to talk about smart drugs: cognitive enhancers like hydergine, piracetam and deprenyl—different drugs that are commonly prescribed for senile dementia, but have been used by people to enhance their memory or improve their concentration. He didn't seem to be very open to even discussing the research or hearing anything about it. He kept cutting us off, and he'd talk about how dangerous methamphetamine was, how this was sending the wrong message to people and how the whole idea of putting "smart" before "drugs" was wrong, and there was no smart way to use drugs. He would not even carefully consider what we were saying; he had his mind made up. And what I think was so interesting is that since he's developed multiple sclerosis and has had to use medical marijuana to treat the symptoms of this disorder, he's now become one of the leading spokespeople for the legalization of medical marijuana. What is it about illness that turns people around? People think that medical marijuana is a joke until they're faced with an illness, or until a loved one is, and then they really understand the medical value that it has and what a horrible, horrible atrocity it is that it's against the law.

DAMON: Is there a primary goal of your work or a primary message you're trying to get out?

DAVID: It seemed to me since I was a child that our species is in ecological danger, destroying ourselves. Since I was a teenager, since my very first psychedelic experiences, I felt a very strong commitment to help elevate and expand consciousness on this planet through my work. I made a personal pact with what I felt was DNA or higher intelligence. I felt that if I aligned my personal mission with life's overall mission, then I would always be supported throughout my life in what I was doing, and I would be working for a noble cause.

DAMON: And what is DNA trying to do?

DAVID: I think DNA is ultimately trying to create a world where the imagination is externalized, where the mind and the external world become synchronized as one, so that basically whatever we can imagine can become a reality. Literally. And I think that everything throughout our entire evolution has been moving slowly toward that goal. In the past couple thousand years, it's been very steady. And through nanotechnology, through artificial intelligence, through advanced robotics, I think we're entering into an age where we'll be able to control matter with our thoughts and actually be able to create anything that our minds can conceive of. We're very quickly heading into a time where machines are going to be more intelligent than we are, and we're going to most likely merge, I think, with these intelligent machines and develop capacities and abilities that we can barely imagine right now, such as the ability to self-transform. What we can do with computers—digital technology, the way we can morph things on a computer screen—is the beginning of understanding that that's how reality itself is organized, that we can do that with physical reality through nanotechnology and artificial intelligence, that the digital nature of reality itself will allow us to externalize whatever we think. So I think that eventually reality will become like a computer graphic screen, and we'll be able to create whatever we want. That sound right? [Laughs.]

Damon Orion's work has appeared in publications like *Spirituality & Health,* the *MAPS Bulletin, Revolver, High Times, The Wave, Common Ground, Austin Monthly,* and *Massage Magazine* as well as in such webzines as *Reality Sandwich, Acceler8or,* and *New Realities.* His past interviewees include Ram Dass, Oprah Winfrey, Burning Man founder Larry Harvey, Bill Cosby, Rob Brezsny, Cheech and Chong, and members of the Doors, the Grateful Dead, and Jane's Addiction. See damonorion.wordpress.com.

Recommended Reading

Arthur, J. D. *Salvia Divinorum: Doorway to Thought-Free Awareness.* Rochester, Vt.: Park Street Press, 2010. (Originally titled *Peopled Darkness.*)

Brown, David Jay. *Brainchild.* Las Vegas: New Falcon Publications, 1988.

———. *Conversations on the Edge of the Apocalypse.* New York: Palgrave Macmillan, 2005.

———. *Mavericks of Medicine.* Reno: Smart Publications, 2006.

———. *Psychedelic Drug Research: A Comprehensive Review.* New York: Reality Sandwich, 2012.

———. *Virus: The Alien Strain.* Las Vegas: New Falcon Publications, 1999.

Brown, David Jay, and Garry Gordon. *Detox with Oral Chelation.* Reno, Nev.: Smart Publications, 2007.

Brown, David Jay, and Rebecca McClen Novick. *Mavericks of the Mind.* Santa Cruz, Calif.: MAPS, 2010.

———. *Voices from the Edge.* Santa Cruz, Calif.: Crossing Press, 1995.

Bryanton, Rob. *Imagining the Tenth Dimension.* Bloomington, Ind.: Trafford Publishing, 2007.

Budden, Albert. *Electric UFOs: Fireballs, Electromagnetics and Abnormal States.* New York: Sterling Publishing, 1998.

Chapkis, Wendy. *Dying to Get High: Marijuana as Medicine.* New York: NYU Press, 2008.

Dobkin de Rios, Marlene, and Oscar Janiger. *LSD, Spirituality, and the Creative Process.* Rochester, Vt.: Park Street Press, 2003.

Fadiman, James. *The Psychedelic Explorer's Guide: Safe, Therapeutic, and Sacred Journeys.* Rochester, Vt.: Park Street Press, 2011.

Graboi, Nina. *One Foot in the Future: A Woman's Spiritual Journey.* Santa Cruz, Calif.: Aerial Press, 2000.

Grinspoon, Lester. *Marihuana Reconsidered.* San Francisco: Quick American Archives, 1994.

Harpur, Patrick. *Daimonic Reality.* Enumclaw, Wa.: Pine Winds Press, 2003.

Herbert, Nick. *Elemental Mind: Human Consciousness and the New Physics.* New York: Plume, 1994.

James, William. *The Varieties of the Religious Experience: A Study in Human Nature.* New York: Penguin Classics, 1982.

Jenson, Karl. *Ketamine: Dreams and Realities.* Santa Cruz, Calif.: MAPS, 2004.

Kaku, Michio. *Hyperspace.* Oxford, England: Oxford University Press, 1995.

Kleefeld, Carolyn Mary. *Soul Seeds: Revelations and Drawings.* New York: Cross-Cultural Communications, 2008.

———. *Psyche of Mirrors: A Promenade of Portraits.* New York: Cross-Cultural Communications & The Seventh Quarry Press, 2012.

Kurzweil, Ray. *How to Create a Mind: The Secret of Human Thought Revealed.* New York: Viking, 2012.

LaBerge, Stephen, and Howard Rheingold. *Exploring the World of Lucid Dreaming.* New York: Ballantine Books, 1991.

Leary, Timothy. *Info-Psychology.* Las Vegas: New Falcon Publications, 1994.

Lilly, John C. *Programming and Metaprogramming in the Human Biocomputer.* New York: Three Rivers Press/Julian Press, 1987.

Lynch, Gary, and Richard Granger. *Big Brain: The Origins and Future of Human Intelligence.* New York: Palgrave Macmillan, 2009.

Mack, John. *Abduction: Human Encounters with Aliens.* New York: Scribner, 2007.

McKenna, Terence. *The Archaic Revival.* New York: HarperCollins, 1992.

Meldrum, Jeff. *Sasquatch: Legend Meets Science.* New York: Forge Books, 2007.

Narby, Jeremy. *The Cosmic Serpent: DNA and the Origins of Knowledge.* New York: Jeremy P. Tarcher/Putnam, 1999.

Pickover, Clifford A. *Sex, Drugs, Einstein, and Elves.* Reno, Nev.: Smart Publications, 2005.

Radin, Dean. *The Conscious Universe: The Scientific Truth of Psychic Phenomena.* San Francisco: HarperOne, 2009.

Ridley, Matt. *The Rational Optimist: How Prosperity Evolves.* New York: Harper Perennial, 2011.

Siegel, Ronald K. *Intoxication: The Universal Drive for Mind-Altering Substances.* Rochester, Vt.: Park Street Press, 2005.

Sheldrake, Rupert. *Dogs That Know When Their Owners Are Coming Home.* New York: Broadway, 2011.

———. *The Sense of Being Stared At and Other Aspects of the Extended Mind.* New York: Random House, 2004.

Strassman, Rick. *DMT: The Spirit Molecule.* Rochester, Vt.: Park Street Press, 2000.

Turner, D. M. *Salvinorin: The Psychedelic Essence of Salvia Divinorum.* San Francisco: Panther Press, 1996.

Wilson, Robert Anton. *Cosmic Trigger.* Las Vegas: New Falcon Publications, 2008.

About the Author

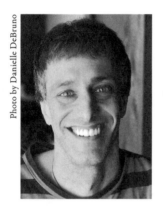

Photo by Danielle DeBruno

David Jay Brown is the coauthor of four best-selling volumes of interviews with leading-edge thinkers, *Mavericks of the Mind, Voices from the Edge, Conversations on the Edge of the Apocalypse,* and *Mavericks of Medicine.* He is also the author of two science-fiction novels, *Brainchild* and *Virus: The Alien Strain,* and is the coauthor of the health science book *Detox with Oral Chelation.* David holds a master's degree in psychobiology from New York University and was responsible for the California-based research in two of British biologist Rupert Sheldrake's books on unexplained phenomena in science: *Dogs That Know When Their Owners Are Coming Home* and *The Sense of Being Stared At.* His work has appeared in numerous magazines, including *Wired, Discover,* and *Scientific American,* and he is periodically the guest editor of the MAPS (Multidisciplinary Association for Psychedelic Studies) *Bulletin.* David writes a popular weekly column for SantaCruzPatch.com called "Catch the Buzz," about cannabis and psychedelic culture, and in 2011 and 2012 he was voted Best Writer in the annual *Good Times* Best of Santa Cruz poll. His news stories have been picked up by *The Huffington Post* and *CBS News.* To find out more about David's work see www.mavericksofthemind.com.

Index